There has been a long-standing recognition of the stress and trauma that reproductive medicine patients may experience [3]. This is reflected in the 2021 American College of Obstetricians and Gynecologists (ACOG) committee opinion recommending that all obstetricians and gynecologists adopt a trauma-informed model of care [4]. There is also an increasing focus on the need to support the mental health of healthcare teams [2]. However, the integration of TIC practices into reproductive medicine clinics has not yet been adequately addressed. This book, *Trauma-Informed Care in Reproductive Medicine*, represents a pioneering effort to compile the latest research, insights, and practical applications of TIC in this specialized field in order to facilitate the critical next step of implementing TIC in the field of reproductive medicine.

This book is geared toward reproductive healthcare professionals and staff, mental health professionals, healthcare administrators, and organizational leaders. While trauma has a global impact, this book is focused primarily on the research and experiences of reproductive medicine patients in the United States. It begins with a broad overview of trauma-informed care and then goes on to focus on a number of specific types of trauma that are likely to impact reproductive patients, including reproductive loss, sexual trauma, medical trauma, trauma perpetrated on individuals due to their sexual orientation or gender expression/identity, racial trauma or discrimination, and paramilitary trauma. The final chapters of this book are tailored for medical professionals, healthcare administrators, and mental health professionals, providing recommendations on how to incorporate trauma-informed care into their respective roles within the healthcare team.

We hope that this book will serve as a valuable resource for medical professionals, mental health professionals, healthcare administrators, and organizational leadership in reproductive medicine and beyond. By integrating and championing trauma-informed care, we can better support the diverse needs of our patients, promote healing and well-being, and ultimately contribute to a more inclusive and responsive healthcare system.

References

1. Gerber MR (editor). Trauma-informed healthcare approaches: a guide for primary care. Springer; 2019.
2. Substance Abuse and Mental Health Services Administration. SAMHSA's Concept of Truama and Guidance for a Trauma-Informed Approach. In: (Vol. HHS Publication No. (SMA) 14-4884). Rockville, MD: Substance Abuse and Mental Health Services Administration; 2014.
3. Jaffe J. Reproductive trauma: psychotherapy with clients experiencing infertility and pregnancy loss. 2nd ed. American Psychological Association; 2024.
4. American College of Obstetricians and Gynecologists, & Committee on Health Care for Underserved Women. Caring for patients who have experienced trauma: ACOG Committee opinion, number 825. Obstet Gynecol 2021;137(4):e94–e99.

Chicago, IL, USA — Angela Lawson
Skokie, IL, USA — Amelia Swanson

Preface

The concept of the provision of trauma-informed care (TIC) to healthcare patients has been adopted in a growing number of healthcare settings, including mental health centers, substance use treatment centers, primary care clinics, and pediatric care facilities [1]. TIC is based on the understanding that exposure to traumatic events (i.e., physical, sexual, and/or psychological) by patients before or during receipt of medical care is unfortunately common and is associated with medical and emotional consequences which may be intensified in the setting of uninformed medical care. The provision of effective TIC from an organizational, as well as individual, perspective provides a safe, nonjudgmental, and collaborative environment in which patients are supported in their healing processes [2]. Trauma-informed care is thus an example of patient-centered care in action.

It is well known that exposure to traumatic events can impact an individual's health, lifestyle choices, behaviors, emotions, and interactions with friends, family, and healthcare professionals [2]. For many people, especially those who have experienced one or more traumatic events, their engagement in medical treatment that is associated with a loss of sense of control (particularly of one's body, future, and/or safety) may result in heightened distress and unwelcome reminders of prior traumatic experiences. This is particularly true for those undergoing fertility treatment as it can be complicated by additional losses and trauma, a sense of emotional and bodily vulnerability, and loss of control. Understanding patients' perceptions and experiences of reproductive care from a trauma-informed lens can help healthcare professionals understand and respond to patients' distress in a supportive manner.

The provision of trauma-informed care also benefits healthcare professionals and staff. Working with a patient population like reproductive medicine patients who are often highly distressed and who have likely experienced prior trauma may be especially difficult for healthcare professionals and staff with their own history of trauma. The ongoing work of supporting reproductive medicine patients through new losses and grief can be emotionally draining for healthcare professionals and staff. Trauma-informed models of care recognize the risk of burnout and vicarious traumatization of healthcare teams and thus include a focus on structural changes to support healthcare professionals and staff so that they can effectively take care of themselves while taking care of patients.

Editors
Angela Lawson
Obstetrics and Gynecology
Northwestern Medicine
Chicago, IL, USA

Amelia Swanson
Licensed Clinical Psychologist
Health Psychology Associates of Illinois PLLC
Skokie, IL, USA

ISBN 978-3-031-67473-0 ISBN 978-3-031-67474-7 (eBook)
https://doi.org/10.1007/978-3-031-67474-7

This Springer imprint is published by the registered company Springer Nature Switzerland AG
The registered company address is: Gewerbestrasse 11, 6330 Cham, Switzerland

Angela Lawson • Amelia Swanson
Editors

Trauma-Informed Reproductive Healthcare

Springer

Trauma-Informed Reproductive Healthcare

Contents

1 **Introduction** 1
Amelia Swanson and Angela Lawson

2 **Trauma-Informed Care in the Setting of Pregnancy Loss** 17
Chloe Warlick and Susan C. Klock

3 **Trauma-Informed Care in Patients with a History of Sexual Trauma** 29
Aisha Kazi and Angela Lawson

4 **Trauma-Informed Care in Patients with a History of Medical Trauma** 39
Amelia Swanson and Krithika Malhotra

5 **Trauma-Informed Care in the Reproductive Clinical Setting for LGBTQ+ Patients** 53
Colin B. Russell, Nicholas S. Raja, and Molly B. Moravek

6 **Trauma-Informed Care for Patients Who Have Experienced Racial Trauma or Discrimination** 67
Danielle A. Kaplan

7 **Trauma-Informed Care: Strategies for Medical Professionals in the Reproductive Endocrinology and Infertility Clinic** 85
Julie Bindeman and Vickie Schafer

8 **Strategies for Clinic Administrators and Staff** 101
Erika L. Kelley

9 **The Role of the Mental Health Professional** 115
Teni Davoudian

10 Special Considerations for Military Personnel, Veterans, and First Responders 129
Erika L. Kelley and Angela Lawson

Index 139

Chapter 1
Introduction

Amelia Swanson and Angela Lawson

Patients receiving care in reproductive endocrinology and infertility (REI) clinics are often highly emotionally distressed. Research shows that as many as 50% or more infertility and fertility preservation patients report experiencing clinically significant symptoms of anxiety and/or depression as a result of their experiences of infertility, pregnancy loss, and other reproductive-related experiences [1–3]. REI patients' distress is often present at the onset of fertility treatment, worsens after failed treatment cycles, can lead to premature treatment termination, can persist during the course of a healthy pregnancy and after the birth of a healthy child, and may be comparable to the distress seen in newly diagnosed cancer patients [1, 4–6]. Infertility and pregnancy loss have also been found to be experienced by many patients as traumatic with patients experiencing a loss of sense of control over their bodies and their futures [7]. Although it may be hypothesized that infertility or pregnancy loss may reflect the first potentially traumatic event faced by the stereotypical young high socioeconomic status fertility patient, it is likely that most REI patients have previously been exposed to other potentially traumatic events (see, e.g., [8]) and that infertility, pregnancy loss, and other negative reproductive experiences may be emotionally triggering of past traumatic experiences. The false assumption that REI patients are "only" struggling to cope with infertility or that infertility and loss are not potentially traumatizing may lead to biased assumptions by clinic teams as to REI patients' interpersonal presentation; patients may be experienced by clinic staff as needy, anxious, demanding, angry and the like when in fact they are not "difficult patients" rather they are traumatized patients in need of empathy and

A. Swanson (✉)
Health Psychology Associates of Illinois PLLC, Skokie, IL, USA
e-mail: amelia@healthpsychologyillinois.com

A. Lawson
Obstetrics and Gynecology, Northwestern Medicine, Chicago, IL, USA
e-mail: alawsonphd@gmail.com

A. Lawson, A. Swanson (eds.), *Trauma-Informed Reproductive Healthcare*,
https://doi.org/10.1007/978-3-031-67474-7_1

support. Inadvertent invalidation of patients' emotional distress with unrealistic assurances of future treatment success, blaming patients for their infertility or other reproductive experiences due to stress or other concerns, lack of ongoing assessment of emotional well-being and experience of trauma, lack of provision of emotional support and referrals to qualified mental health professionals or support groups, lack of encouragement of patient engagement in shared decision-making, clinic design which focuses on a narrow demographic patient population, and other non-trauma aware aspects of REI care are the opposite of patient-centered care and risk further harming REI patients [9–11].

Trauma-informed care (TIC) is a concept that has grown in national importance and recognition over the last 10 years and is a model for the application of effective patient-centered care and support to patients. The Substance Abuse and Mental Health Services Administration (SAMHSA) has published documents to define trauma and provide recommendations for TIC implementation for healthcare organizations. Although the American College of Obstetricians and Gynecologists (ACOG) has published guidelines for TIC [12], at the time of publication of this book the American Society for Reproductive Medicine (ASRM), had not yet published guidelines or recommendations for TIC and there is limited research or published material on TIC in the reproductive medicine population.

While TIC aims to support all patients, it can also benefit healthcare professionals and staff [13]. Lack of control within one's work environment, imbalanced demands and resources, and unaddressed trauma in medical teams and staff are primary causes of burnout. TIC practices help address this and therefore can reduce burnout and improve well-being for patients, staff, and healthcare professionals alike [14]. This chapter will introduce the concepts of trauma, trauma-informed care, and special considerations of trauma-informed care in reproductive medicine.

Trauma

The concept of trauma is vast and complex with no one agreed upon definition. This likely contributes to the frequent non-clinical use of the words "traumatic," "traumatizing," "triggered," and "triggering" when an individual experiences a wide range of difficult life experiences that are typically not associated with trauma responses [15]. However, some of the more commonly used definitions of trauma come from the American Psychiatric Association's Diagnostic and Statistical Manual (DSM-5) [16] and SAMHSA [17]. Some common themes across definitions are that trauma is an emotional response to one or more discrete, ongoing, and/or chronic events that may be perceived to be life-threatening, include perceived risk or actual experience of physical or sexual violence/injury, and/or are highly emotionally disturbing. By this definition, the experience of a traumatic event(s) threatens an individual's sense of safety (physical or emotional) or integrity, and perception of the event can vary and is a crucial factor in making a specific experience traumatizing to an individual. Experiencing one or more traumatic events that the individual perceives to be traumatizing increases the risk of the development of posttraumatic stress disorder and other symptoms of psychological distress such as anxiety and low mood [16].

The DSM-5 is the diagnostic manual used by mental health practitioners to aid in the assessment and assignment of mental health diagnoses. Under the DSM-5 definition of posttraumatic stress disorder (PTSD), a traumatic event is identified as an event that may be directly experienced, witnessed, learned about (e.g., learning about a loved one who has been exposed to a traumatic event), or experienced through occupational aversive exposure(s). Prior to the DSM's identification of PTSD as a mental health disorder, the symptoms associated with PTSD had been documented in civilians as early as the nineteenth century who had been exposed to catastrophic events and military personnel during the Civil War [18, 19]. However, the DSM's concept of trauma and PTSD was based on the experience of military veterans exposed to discrete traumatic events that happened in the course of war [19, 20]. Referred to as "shell shock" or "combat fatigue," it was not until after the Vietnam War that PTSD was included as a formal diagnosis in the DSM-III. The definition of trauma has expanded since the publication of the DSM-III based on critiques and advances in research to capture a vast array of possible events that could be trauma-inducing to both soldiers and civilians. Over time, the definition of trauma has extended beyond the mere experience of a catastrophic event(s) that risks the development of psychiatric distress to include understanding of how trauma responses are incited by such events. It is now generally accepted that from a psychological perspective, the perception and appraisal of an event are crucial aspects of the experience of trauma [17].

From a biological perspective, in the presence of a perceived threatening event(s) the thalamus is believed to triage sensory input to determine what other areas of the brain need to be activated in response to the aversive event(s). The thalamus provides information to both the hippocampus and the amygdala with the hippocampus aiding in memory formation and the amygdala generating an emotional valence to the exposure and preparing for potential threat via activation of the sympathetic nervous system to engage in the fight, flight, freeze, or faint acute stress response [21, 22]. Finally, upon exposure to potentially threatening stimuli, the prefrontal cortex is believed to play a role in decision-making related to which cognitive and/or emotional responses should follow the exposure. The PTSD symptoms of re-experiencing, avoidance, negative alterations in thoughts and feelings, and alterations in arousal and reactivity are thought to be in part caused by hyperactivation/hyperregulation of normal fear and survival processes which affect memory, attention, and emotions. For example, over-activation of the amygdala in the context of under-activation of the prefrontal cortex may be implicated in the experience of the PTSD symptoms of re-experiencing and hyperarousal (e.g., hypervigilance, an exaggerated startle response, irritability), whereas under-activation of the hippocampus and prefrontal cortex is believed to play a role in the experience of dissociation/numbing, avoidance, recurrent intrusive memories and nightmares, flashbacks, and altered cognitions [22, 23]. It should also be noted that there are non-biologic responses to exposure to potentially traumatizing experiences that are reflective of the individual's internal or external coping strategies (e.g., appeasement) [24].

Like the DSM-5 definition, SAMHSA's definition of trauma is inclusive of many types of trauma and is defined as resulting "from an event, series of events, or set of circumstances that is experienced by an individual as physically or emotionally harmful or life-threatening and that has lasting adverse effects on the individual's functioning and mental, physical, social, emotional, or spiritual well-being" ([17], p. 7). Both the DSM-5 and SAMHSA focus not just on traumatic events but also on the individual's subjective experience of the event(s) and the sequelae of being exposed to the event(s). SAMHSA uses the concept of "the 3 E's of trauma" (event(s), experience of event(s), and effect) to define the different aspects that may make an event traumatic. Different aversive events may lead to trauma, including actual or threatened physical or psychological harms or extreme neglect of a child. SAMHSA uses the DSM-5's definition of trauma to clarify *events* that may be traumatic such as physical abuse, sexual abuse, threats of violence, accidents, catastrophic weather events, mass shootings, emotional/psychological abuse, and neglect of a child. The *experience* of the event by the individual is an important component as well, as two people experiencing the same event may associate different meaning to the event and have different emotional reactions. The experience of an event may also be influenced by culture, social support, developmental stage, and other factors. The final E, *effect*, is about the long-lasting impact that the traumatic event has on an individual and their development. This effect may be immediate, delayed, short-term, or long-term. Some of the effects of trauma may be visible and notable, including agitation, anxiety, depression, irritability, mood swings, being easily startled, hypervigilance, flashbacks or re-experiencing, difficulty concentrating, self-blame, guilt or shame, feeling numb, difficulty trusting others, avoiding medical procedures or care, indirect or unclear communication, and/or freezing or fainting. Other effects may not be visible and may be neurobiological and can impact an individual's long-term health as well as the health and well-being of their children and grandchildren [25, 26].

Prevalence of Trauma

Exposure to traumatic events is prevalent, with some studies showing that almost 90% of people in the U.S. report experiencing at least one potentially traumatic event which could qualify under DSM-5 criteria [27]. Exposure to trauma often begins in childhood and there is a growing body of research that has connected the experience of childhood trauma with adult mental and physical health problems. Adverse childhood events (ACEs) are potentially traumatic childhood events such as: physical abuse, sexual abuse, verbal abuse, physical neglect, emotional neglect, family member with a mental illness, family member with addiction, family member in prison, witnessing intimate partner violence, and losing a parent to separation, divorce, or death [28]. ACEs are unfortunately common, with 61% of adults reporting at least one ACE, and 16% reporting four or more ACEs. Additionally, women, multiracial, Black, Hispanic, lesbian, gay, and bisexual individuals have been reported to be at greater risk for experiencing more ACEs. People with 4 or more ACEs have been found to have a higher risk of stroke, asthma, COPD, cancer, kidney disease, diabetes, obesity, depression, smoking, and heavy drinking [8]. There is no rigorous research indicating that ACEs are biologically related to infertility or pregnancy loss, although some of the known health consequences of trauma exposure may damage fertility such as smoking, heavy alcohol use, obesity, and diabetes among other consequences.

Trauma exposure is of course not limited to childhood and adults are at risk of exposure to numerous traumatic events. For example, rates of sexual abuse and assault as well as intimate partner violence are high, and researchers believe that reported rates are likely underestimates of true occurrences. Some U.S. studies have found that as many as 30% of girls and 16% of boys have experienced childhood sexual abuse. Among adults surveyed in the U.S. National Intimate Partner and Sexual Violence Survey, at least 44% of women and 25% of men report having experienced contact sexual violence [29]; sexual harassment and racial, identity, and sexual orientation harassment/violence are also common [30–33]. Rates of intimate partner violence (IPV) in the U.S. are also high with about 36% of women and 29% of men reporting experiencing physical forms of these behaviors; psychological IPV is even more common than physical IPV and is equally emotionally damaging [34]. Research similarly finds the global prevalence of violence and harassment to be problematic (see, e.g., [35, 36]) and infertility is believed to be a risk factor for IPV [37]. The high rates of sexual assault, abuse, harassment, and other adverse exposures mean that many fertility patients may have a history of sexual and other trauma; fertility treatment may be a reminder of that trauma due to frequent pelvic exams, the power or identity differential between the patient and their healthcare professional, a feeling of loss of control related to a diagnosis of infertility or pregnancy loss, and/or transvaginal ultrasounds and other invasive procedures. The frequency of exposure to aversive events also highlights the need for a trauma-informed healthcare treatment approach that realizes the prevalence and consequences of traumatic events, recognizes the signs and symptoms of trauma, responds to patients by providing appropriate support, and avoids re-traumatizing them.

Trauma-Informed Care

In light of the high probability that (1) the majority of people in the U.S. and throughout the world have experienced one or more potentially traumatic events, (2) the low probability that they have been assessed by their healthcare team for such histories [38], (3) the known medical and emotional risks of trauma exposure, and (4) the risk of re-traumatization during receipt of medical care and more specifically fertility care, patient-centered care which attends to these concerns is necessary. Trauma-informed care is such an approach to patient care that is reflected in all levels of an organization and focuses not only on screening for and treating the consequences of trauma but also recognizes the importance of appropriate care in all patient encounters. The application of a universal approach to patient care that recognizes the high risk of trauma exposure benefits not only the well-being of patients but also of healthcare professionals and staff.

Benefits of TIC to Patients and REI Clinic Teams

Medical staff and healthcare professionals are reporting increasing rates of burnout and are leaving the profession, especially since the beginning of the COVID-19 pandemic [39]. While burnout, compassion fatigue, and vicarious trauma are the most common concepts of stress discussed in relation to healthcare professionals and staff, many may also be experiencing traumatic stress. Work in healthcare may expose individuals to potentially traumatic events and/or may be re-traumatizing for staff and healthcare professionals with prior trauma exposure or current non-work related trauma [13, 14]. Workplaces that value and implement effective TIC not only provide appropriate care to patients but also to healthcare professionals and staff through efforts to protect and support employees exposed to patient trauma as well as engagement in SAMHSA's 6 principles of TIC (trust and transparency, collaboration, choice, safety, peer support, and awareness of cultural, historical, and gender issues) as applied to employees. In the context of REI clinics, trauma-informed organizations recognize the unique and shared potential traumas of their patient population(s) (e.g., pregnancy loss) as well as the risks of employee exposure to such potential traumatizing experiences and respond by balancing organizational resources and demands while also promoting staff well-being. The application of TIC to healthcare professionals and teams may provide an increased sense of control which can lead to greater efficacy in their job. Additionally, some studies have shown that TIC implementation improved organizational climate and staff retention in a medical setting [40, 41].

TIC for patients and healthcare teams begins at the organizational level and involves all levels and people in an organization; all of whom should receive ongoing TIC training and assessment of effective application of TIC strategies. Within the context of REI clinics, SAMHSA's four guiding assumptions of trauma-informed organizations (the four "R's") [17] can be interpreted within the context of REI clinics to mean clinics which (1) *realize* the widespread effect of trauma and the likely exposure of REI patients (and staff) to past and current trauma, (2) *recognize* the signs and symptoms of trauma in patients (e.g., patient distress in ultrasounds following pregnancy loss) and healthcare teams (e.g., burnout, distress related to non-work related trauma exposure), (3) *respond* to both patients and healthcare teams with appropriate non-judgmental support (e.g., recognizing how difficult it may be to receive a negative pregnancy result) as well as the integration of trauma-related knowledge into organization policy and procedures, and (4) understand the potential paths for recovery from trauma as well as potential paths for *re-traumatization*.

SAMHSA's six principles of TIC used by trauma-informed organizations (safety, trust and transparency, collaboration, choice, peer support, and awareness of cultural, historical, and gender issues) [17] are highly applicable in the context of REI care. REI patients and staff alike should have an actual and perceived sense of ***safety*** while receiving care or working in the clinic. This includes physical safety as well as psychological safety. In a fertility clinic, this could mean having a layout of clinic spaces that provides patients with privacy and safety (e.g., exam table not facing the door or window, easy access to the consult room door by patient and staff, presence of diverse artwork and gender-neutral clinic forms, respectful communication about patient needs/identity, and procedure suites and phlebotomy spaces that provide sound barriers to hearing other patient's care or conversations). Another example of safety would include staff feeling safe to communicate to leadership any potential issues without fear of being dismissed or retaliated against.

It is also important for an REI clinic to show ***trustworthiness and transparency*** to both patients and staff. Examples of trustworthiness and transparency could include clinics that are upfront and clear about any errors made in scheduling or care with a concrete plan to prevent the same issue in the future. Other examples include the communication of organizational decisions early and clearly to staff to increase staff trust in the organization, setting realistic treatment expectations for patients, and use of empathy and emotionally validating language with patients and REI teams.

Peer support is another key principle for TIC but one which may not be present in some REI clinics. Support for patients by others who have had similarly difficult experiences (e.g., infertility or loss) can help patients feel support, hope, and promote resilience and healing [17]. In an REI clinic, this could include a support group facilitated at the clinic, or a clinic having a robust referral process to outside support groups or other emotional support resources. Studies have shown that fertility patients may experience similar levels of stress as cancer patients (see, e.g., [1]), yet fertility patients often have less institutional and social support. For example, anecdotally many cancer centers have embedded psychosocial oncology services that include individual psychotherapy and support groups, but most fertility clinics do not have mental health support embedded in their clinic [42].

SAMHSA's principal of ***collaboration and mutuality*** focuses on reducing the power differential within the organization as well as between healthcare professionals and patients to allow both patients and staff to share questions and concerns, engage in shared decision-making, and develop healing and respectful professional relationships. In this sense, every member of an REI clinic team (e.g., physicians, nurses, mental health professionals, ultrasonographers, phlebotomists, scheduling teams, administrative staff, lab teams, custodial staff, etc.) plays a crucial role in ongoing clinic culture and the provision of patient care by modeling healthy, respectful, and supportive relationships.

Trauma-informed REI clinics should also encourage ***empowerment, voice, and choice*** from all organization members and from patients. Part of this principle is recognizing the ability of patients to heal and recover from trauma and REI teams should be leaders and active collaborators in that process. In an REI clinic, staff should encourage and support patients in advocating for their needs, asking questions about medical and other decisions and outcomes, and making their treatment needs and priorities part of the medical decision-making process. We recognize that clinic teams have limited time to interact with patients and that the encouragement of questions and patient advocacy takes time not always readily available in an already hectic daily clinic schedule. However, the failure of organizations to support clinics in meeting this TIC principal risks harming patients and healthcare professionals alike by continuing a model of care which reinforces a paternalistic power differential between patients and healthcare teams that invalidates patients as deserving, active, and important participants in their own care. Further, REI clinic leadership should also support staff in advocating for their own needs and provide sufficient organizational support for staff to effectively and safely perform their work responsibilities.

Finally, it is important for REI clinics to recognize and avoid further harm associated with ***cultural, historical, and gender issues*** (e.g., stereotypes and biases) that negatively affect patients as well as clinic staff and leadership. Ongoing organizational provision of training and policies that support culturally informed care, responsive diversity and inclusion practices for all organizational members, recognition of the historical and ongoing harm caused to minoritized groups by healthcare professionals and systems (e.g., forced sterilization, medical experimentation, discrimination against LGBTQ+ patients), awareness of historical gender-biases and experiences (e.g., infertility inaccurately portrayed as a woman's fault, victim blaming women for their experience of trauma and infertility, invalidation of women's pain, and risk of sexual victimization) are vital. Reproductive medical society guidance highlights the importance of not discriminating against patients based on their identity and other factors (see e.g., [43]). REI clinics should continue efforts to improve equal access to care and treatment outcomes for patients who are often under-represented in medicine and reproductive endocrinology [44].

Special Consideration for TIC in REI Clinics

There are numerous aspects of medical care that occur in the context of REI clinics which are relevant to the provision of effective TIC at the organizational and patient level. Although not all of these aspects of care are unique to REI patients and clinics, the unique combination of these factors may pose increased emotional risks to patients and REI clinic teams (see Fig. 1.1).

Highly Distressed Patient Population It seems logical that most if not all REI patients would prefer not to have to use fertility treatments to grow their families. For example, infertility patients have often been trying to grow their family for a year or longer without success and potentially with pregnancy loss experiences prior to initial consultation in an REI clinic. The diagnosis of infertility, pregnancy loss, and other aversive reproductive experiences are associated with risk of patient

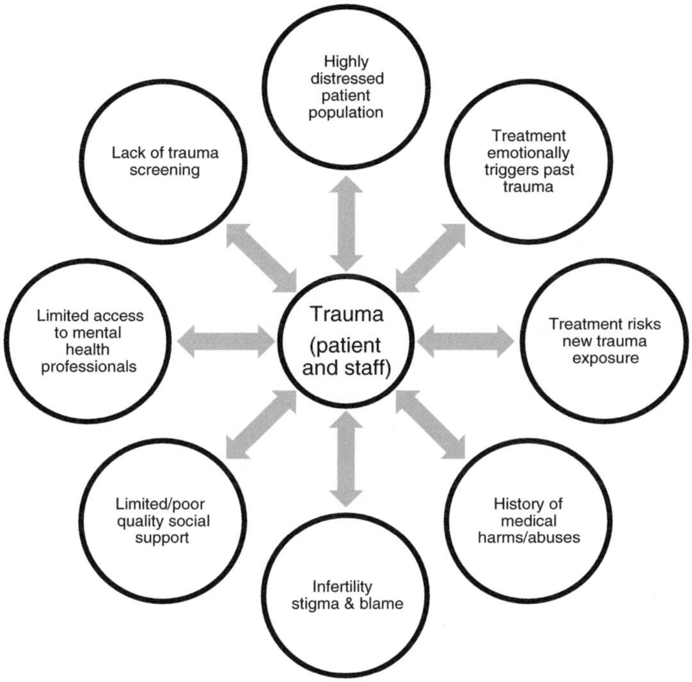

Fig. 1.1 Factors impacting trauma for fertility patients and REI teams

distress [7]. As previously discussed, high levels of psychological distress have been noted in patients upon initiation of fertility treatment, throughout the course of fertility treatment, during the course of a health pregnancy and after the birth of a healthy child, and this distress may lead to premature treatment termination [1, 2, 5, 6]. The worsening of patient distress during the course of fertility treatments not only poses psychological risk to patients but also to the healthcare teams working to support them. Compassion fatigue, burnout, and vicarious traumatization via chronic exposure to patient traumas are of particular concern for those working in REI clinics. Dual efforts to provide empathic support to patients and clinic team members are necessary in the provision of TIC.

Focus on Sexual Behavior, Repeated Invasive and Potentially Painful Exams, Needle and Sedation Exposure, and Risk of Medical Trauma Given the high risk of being sexually victimized as child and/or as an adult it would be expected that the focus in REI care on sexual behavior, STI history, vaginal and other invasive exams conducted by someone with greater power and control than the patient would likely be emotionally difficult for many REI patients. These experiences could trigger memories of being assaulted (or other trauma exposures) and heighten patients' emotional distress. Further, patients who have prior histories of medical trauma may have developed needle, sedation, and other anxieties related to medical procedures.

Fertility care also exposes patients to risk of medical trauma resulting from events such as ovarian torsion, ovarian hyperstimulation syndrome, ectopic pregnancies, pregnancy loss, and emergency or unexpected surgeries (e.g., oophorectomy, salpingectomy, hysterectomy, TESE). Awareness of patients' histories of trauma, of the ability for aspects of medical care to be re-traumatizing or newly traumatic, that patients' appraisal of events may be traumatic, and of clinic team exposures to chronic aversive experiences can be useful in providing supportive medical care and referrals to mental health professionals and peer groups.

History of Discrimination, Abuse, Disparate Access to Care, Disparate Outcomes, Invalidation of Women's Experience of Pain, Fertility Fraud, and Reproductive Errors The history of obstetrics and gynecology is plagued by horrific atrocities committed against Black and Brown women including surgeries without sedation, forced sterilization, and the like [45]. There continues to be disparate treatment of minoritized women who have been identified as having disparate access to and outcomes of fertility treatment [44]. Other individuals have also been discriminated against in fertility clinics including the refusal of some clinics to treat LGBTQ+ individuals or single people [43]. Further, in light of the historical invalidation of women's pain associated with reproductive concerns (e.g., endometriosis) [46] and numerous publicized instances of fertility fraud and REI clinic errors, it is unsurprising that many fertility patients may be anxious about how they will be treated in their clinic and whether or not they or their genetic materials are safe in the REI clinic. Implementation of TIC practices is especially important in REI clinics given this history, particularly efforts at transparency and trustworthiness.

Stigma, Victim Blaming, and Lack of Emotional Support for Fertility Patients Infertility and pregnancy loss have historically been viewed as stigmatizing experiences which violate social norms to have children. The experience of stigma is associated with reduced engagement in social support seeking despite evidence which shows that receipt of empathic social support can aid in coping with difficult life events [47]. Although social support can be beneficial for those experiencing infertility, loss and other aversive reproductive experiences; receipt of non-empathetic "support" from social networks and healthcare teams can be damaging and may contribute to REI patients suffering in silence without receipt of much needed support. For example, those who share their experience of infertility or loss may receive unsolicited advice/commentary intended to be well-meaning but which is intensely hurtful (e.g., "maybe you weren't meant to have a baby"), further stigmatizing (e.g., shaming women for their difficulty conceiving or making disparaging comments about men's masculinity), blaming (e.g., "you should just relax and you'll get pregnant"), or which invalidate the patient's desire to have a genetic child or carry a pregnancy (e.g., "you should just adopt"). It may also be emotionally triggering for patients who have directly or indirectly experienced prior stigma, blame, and/or shame associated with prior traumas (e.g., women who have been blamed for what they were wearing or use of alcohol prior to being sexually victimized) if they are again victim blamed (e.g., blaming a patient's stress for the infertility or loss without rigorous research supporting such a relationship), this time for their aversive reproductive experiences [48]. Despite the high level of distress in patients and benefits of social support, few clinics have integrated mental health professionals (MHPs) and few patients receive needed emotional support [2, 42]. The lack of in-clinic MHPs may also serve as a barrier to screening for trauma as lack of professional psychological supports hinders such screening [38].

Limited Screening for Trauma Given that the experience of trauma is widespread, universal screening for trauma is important in all medical clinics including REI. However, research finds that few healthcare professionals, including ObGyns, screen for trauma [38]. Screening for trauma has a number of potential benefits for patients including identifying patients that may benefit from additional support or attention to how their history of trauma may impact their current medical care, helping patients identify how a history of trauma may be impacting their experience at the REI clinic, and it sends a powerful message to patients that the clinic is sensitive and supportive to issues of trauma. Screening for trauma may be challenging for all patients and particularly for REI patients as they may not feel comfortable disclosing their trauma in a setting associated with many potential trauma triggers, they may not recognize their experiences as traumatic, or they may be worried they will be scrutinized or denied treatment due to their distress or history of trauma. It is important for REI teams to recognize that screening will not identify all cases of trauma and that the integration of TIC practices into all levels of the organization is necessary for the development of patient trust.

Unfortunately, there is no one screening tool for trauma that is comprehensive, but there are a number of different tools that can be considered (see, e.g., Table 1.1).

In addition to the integration of screening for psychological distress and trauma history into clinic forms, REI team members should also consider orally asking patients questions relevant to a potential trauma history as patients may not feel comfortable disclosing trauma in written documentation; screening should also occur in a private setting without the patient's partner present. Questions could include: Have any events in your life impacted your health or made you uncomfortable or concerned about seeking medical care? Is there anything I can do to help you feel safer or comfortable during your time in the clinic? Have you ever experienced

Table 1.1 Trauma screeners related to symptoms of PTSD or trauma

Measure	Number of items	Focus of items
PTSD Checklist for DSM-5 (PCL-5) [49]	20	Current symptoms of PTSD
Primary Care–PTSD screener (PC-PTSD-5) [50]	5	Current symptoms of PTSD
Adverse Childhood Experiences Screening Questionnaire for Adults [28]	10	Exposure to aversive events prior to age 18
Life Events Checklist for DSM-5 (LEC-5) [51]	17	Lifetime DSM-5 exposure to Criterion A events

any frightening or traumatic events? Would you like to talk about any of these experiences? REI teams should avoid asking for specifics or details about trauma experiences if they are not relevant or crucial to medical care. Additionally, patients should be screened for strength and resilience too! Ask patients about their strengths, their supports, their goals, and resilience. In asking about patients' supports and resilience, REI teams will have a better understanding of how to support patients in a comprehensive manner as well as communicate to patients that they are confident in their abilities to heal and persevere.

Summary

REI patients enter treatment with pre-existing histories of trauma and are at risk of exposure to new trauma and triggering of past trauma during receipt of fertility care. Despite the understanding that trauma exposure increases the risk of physical, emotional, social, and other concerns, healthcare professionals may not adequately screen patients for a history of past or current trauma or symptoms of PTSD. Failure to screen for trauma, understand the consequences of trauma, and provide universal TIC and adequate emotional support risks harm to patients. Further, the exposure of REI clinic staff to patient trauma as well as staff members' own history of trauma risks harming staff as well. REI clinics would benefit from ongoing education related to TIC, examination of clinic spaces and marketing to ensure patient safety is prioritized, modification of clinic forms and other materials to be supportive of our diverse patient population, encouragement of shared decision-making, engagement in accountability and transparency when errors are made, development of close professional relationships with peer support groups and mental health professionals, and self-reflection as to the ways in which the care being provided could be improved to best support patients.

References

1. Lawson AK, Klock SC, Pavone ME, Hirshfeld-Cytron J, Smith KN, Kazer RR. Prospective study of depression and anxiety in female fertility preservation and infertility patients. Fertil Steril. 2014;102(5):1377–84. https://doi.org/10.1016/j.fertnstert.2014.07.765.
2. Pasch LA, Holley SR, Bleil ME, Shehab D, Katz PP, Adler NE. Addressing the needs of fertility treatment patients and their partners: are they informed of and do they receive mental health services? Fertil Steril. 2016;106(1):209–15. e202. https://doi.org/10.1016/j.fertnstert.2016.03.006.
3. Wang A, Pasch L, Holley S, Huddleston HG, Jaswa EG. Anxiety and depression in patients undergoing oocyte cryopreservation and infertility. Fertil Steril. 2021;116(3):e360.
4. Brandes M, van der Steen JOM, Bodkdam SB, Hamilton CJCM, de Bruin JP, Nelen WLDM, Kremer JAM. When and why do subfertile couples discontinue their fertility care? A longitudinal cohort study in a secondary care subfertility population. Hum Reprod. 2009;24:3127–35.

5. Gameiro S, Boivin J, Peronace L, Verhaak CM. Why do patients discontinue fertility treatment? A systematic review of reasons and predictors of discontinuation in fertility treatment. Hum Reprod Update. 2012;18(6):652–69. https://doi.org/10.1093/humupd/dms031.
6. Oftedal A, Tsotsi S, Kaasen A, Mayerhofer LJK, Roysamb E, Smajlagic D, et al. Anxiety and depression in expectant parents: ART versus spontaneous conception. Hum Reprod. 2023;38(9):1755–60. https://doi.org/10.1093/humrep/dead133.
7. Brigance CA, Kim SR, Kashubeck-West S. Mean comparisons of trauma symptoms between a reproductive trauma sample and a normative sample: toward a trauma-informed practice. Psychol Trauma. 2023; https://doi.org/10.1037/tra0001468.
8. Merrick MT, Ford DC, Ports KA, Guinn AS. Prevalence of adverse childhood experiences from the 2011-2014 behavioral risk factor surveillance system in 23 states. JAMA Pediatr. 2018;172(11):1038–44. https://doi.org/10.1001/jamapediatrics.2018.2537.
9. Institute of Medicine. Crossing the quality chasm: a new health system for the 21st century. Washington, DC: National Academy Press; 2001.
10. Marthi S, Shandley LM, Ismaeel N, Anderson-Bialis J, Anderson-Bialis D, Kawwass JF, et al. Factors associated with a positive experience at US fertility clinics: the male partner perspective. J Assist Reprod Genet. 2023;40(6):1317–28. https://doi.org/10.1007/s10815-023-02848-2.
11. Shandley LM, Hipp HS, Anderson-Bialis J, Anderson-Bialis D, Boulet SL, McKenzie LJ, Kawwass JF. Patient-centered care: factors associated with reporting a positive experience at United States fertility clinics. Fertil Steril. 2020;113(4):797–810. https://doi.org/10.1016/j.fertnstert.2019.12.040.
12. American College of Obstetricians and Gynecologists, & Committee on Health Care for Underserved Women. Caring for patients who have experienced trauma: ACOG Committee opinion, number 825. Obstet Gynecol. 2021;137(4):e94–9.
13. Elisseou S. Trauma-informed care: a missing link in addressing burnout. J Healthc Leadersh. 2023;15:169. https://doi.org/10.2147/JHLS389271.
14. Forrest L, Abdurrahman M, Ritsma A. Recognizing compassion fatigue, vicarious trauma, and burnout. In: Hategan A, Saperson K, Harms S, Waters H, editors. Humanism and resilience in residency training : a guide to physician wellness. Cham, Switzerland: Springer; 2020.
15. Bonilla S, Natarajan M, Koven J, White L, Lamb S. The discourse of being 'triggered': uses and meanings among counselling students. Couns Psychother Res. 2023;23(2):551–62.
16. American Psychiatric Association. Diagnostic and statistical manual of mental disorders. 5th ed. Arlington, VA: American Psychiatric Association; 2013.
17. Substance Abuse and Mental Health Services Administration (2014) SAMHSA's concept of truama and guidance for a trauma-informed approach. In (Vol. HHS Publication No. (SMA) 14–4884). Rockville, MD: Substance Abuse and Mental Health Services Administration.
18. Birmes P, Hatton L, Brunet A, Schmitt L. Early historical literature for post-traumatic symptomatology. Stress Health. 2003;19(1):17–26.
19. Committee on the Assessment of Ongoing Effects in the Treatment of Posttraumatic Stress Disorder, & Institute of Medicine (2012) History, diagnostic criteria, and epidemiology. Treatment for posttraumatic stress disorder in military and veteran populations: initial assessment. Retrieved from https://www.ncbi.nlm.nih.gov/books/NBK201095/
20. Kulka RA, Schlenger WE, Fairbank JA, Hough RL, Jordan BK, Marmar CR, Weiss DS. Trauma and the Vietnam war generation: report of findings from the National Vietnam Veterans Readjustment Study. New York: Brunner/Mazel; 1990.
21. Kozlowska K, Walker P, McLean L, Carrive P. Fear and the defense cascade: clinical implications and management. Harv Rev Psychiatry. 2015;23(4):263–87. https://doi.org/10.1097/HRP.0000000000000065.
22. Weiss SJ. Neurobiological alterations associated with traumatic stress. Perspect Psychiatr Care. 2007;43(3):114–22. https://doi.org/10.1111/j.1744-6163.2007.00120.x.
23. Diamond DM, Zoladz PR. Dysfunctional or hyperfunctional? The amygdala in posttraumatic stress disorder is the bull in the evolutionary China shop. J Neurosci Res. 2016;94(6):437–44. https://doi.org/10.1002/jnr.23684.

24. Fitzgerald LF, Swan S, Fischer K. Why didn't she just report him? The psychological and legal implications of women's responses to sexual harassment. J Soc Issues. 1995;51:117–38.
25. Buss CP, Entringer SP, Moog NKM, Toepfer PM, Fair DAP, Simhan HNMDMS, et al. Intergenerational transmission of maternal childhood maltreatment exposure: implications for fetal brain development. J Am Acad Child Adolesc Psychiatry. 2017;56(5):373–82. https://doi.org/10.1016/j.jaac.2017.03.001.
26. Narayan AJ, Lieberman AF, Masten AS. Intergenerational transmission and prevention of adverse childhood experiences (ACEs). Clin Psychol Rev. 2021;85:101997. https://doi.org/10.1016/j.cpr.2021.101997.
27. Kilpatrick DG, Resnick HS, Milanak ME, Miller MW, Keyes KM, Friedman MJ. National estimates of exposure to traumatic events and PTSD prevalence using DSM-IV and DSM-5 criteria. J Trauma Stress. 2013;26(5):537–47. https://doi.org/10.1002/jts.21848.
28. Felitti VJ, Anda RF, Nordenberg D, Williamson DF, Spitz AM, Edwards V, et al. Relationship of childhood abuse and household dysfunction to many of the leading causes of death in adults. The adverse childhood experiences (ACE) study. Am J Prev Med. 1998;14(4):245–58. https://doi.org/10.1016/s0749-3797(98)00017-8.
29. Smith SG, Zhang X, Basile KC, Merrick MT, Wang J, Kresnow M, Chen J. The National Intimate Partner and Sexual Violence Survey (NISVS): 2015 data brief—updated release. Atlanta, GA: Centers for Disease Control and Prevention; 2018.
30. Bender AK, Lauritsen JL. Violent victimization among lesbian, gay, and bisexual populations in the United States: findings from the National Crime Victimization Survey, 2017-2018. Am J Public Health. 2021;111(2):318–26. https://doi.org/10.2105/AJPH.2020.306017.
31. Bleich SN, Findling MG, Casey LS, Blendon RJ, Benson JM, SteelFisher GK, et al. Discrimination in the United States: experiences of black Americans. Health Serv Res. 2019;54(Suppl 2):1399–408. https://doi.org/10.1111/1475-6773.13220.
32. Fitzgerald LF, Cortina LM. Sexual harassment in work organizations: a view from the 21st century. In: Travis CB, White JW, Rutherford A, Williams WS, Cook SL, Wyche KF, editors. APA handbook of the psychology of women: perspectives on women's private and public lives. Washington, DC: American Psychological Association; 2018. p. 215–34.
33. James SE, Herman JL, Rankin S, Keisling M, Mottet L, Anafi M (2016) The report of the 2015 U.S. transgender survey. Retrieved from Washington, DC.
34. Breiding MJ, Chen J, Black MC. Intimate partner violence in the United States—2010. Atlanta, GA: National Center for Injury Prevention and Control: Centers for Disease Control and Prevention; 2014.
35. Dworkin ER, Krahe B, Zinzow H. The global prevalence of sexual assault: a systematic review of international research since 2010. Psychol Violence. 2021;11(5):497–508. https://doi.org/10.1037/vio0000374.
36. Sardinha L, Maheu-Giroux M, Stockl H, Meyer SR, Garcia-Moreno C. Global, regional, and national prevalence estimates of physical or sexual, or both, intimate partner violence against women in 2018. Lancet. 2022;399(10327):803–13. https://doi.org/10.1016/S0140-6736(21)02664-7.
37. Barishansky SJ, Shapiro P, Meyman G, Pavone ME, Lawson AK. Reproductive endocrinologists' knowledge and attitudes in the identification of intimate partner violence. Fertil Steril. 2021;116(6):1622–30. https://doi.org/10.1016/j.fertnstert.2021.08.011.
38. Farrow VA, Bosch J, Crawford JN, Snead C, Schulkin J. Screening for history of childhood abuse: beliefs, practice patterns, and barriers among obstetrician-gynecologists. Womens Health Issues. 2018;28(6):559–68. https://doi.org/10.1016/j.whi.2018.09.001.
39. Rotenstein LS, Brown R, Sinsky C, Linzer M. The Association of work overload with burnout and intent to leave the job across the healthcare workforce during COVID-19. J Gen Intern Med. 2023;38(8):1920–7. https://doi.org/10.1007/s11606-023-08153-z.
40. Hales TW, Green SA, Bissonette S, Warden A, Diebold J, Koury SP, Nochajski TH. Trauma-informed care outcome study. Res Soc Work Pract. 2019;29(5):529–39.

41. Hales TW, Nochajski TH. A structural regression analysis of trauma-informed climate factors, organizational commitment, and burnout among behavioral healthcare providers in a large public hospital. J Community Psychol. 2020;48(3):777–92. https://doi.org/10.1002/jcop.22292.
42. Woodward JT, Cirino NH, Copland S, Davoudian T. Integrated behavioral health care in reproductive medicine: how and why to include mental health professionals in infertility care teams. Clin Obstet Gynecol. 2024;67(1):222–32. https://doi.org/10.1097/GRF.0000000000000829.
43. Ethics Committee of the American Society for Reproductive Medicine. Access to fertility treatment irrespective of marital status, sexual orientation, or gender identity: an ethics committee opinion. Fertil Steril. 2021;116(2):326–30. https://doi.org/10.1016/j.fertnstert.2021.03.034.
44. Ethics Committee of the American Society for Reproductive Medicine. Electronic address, a. a. o. Disparities in access to effective treatment for infertility in the United States: an ethics committee opinion. Fertil Steril. 2021;116(1):54–63. https://doi.org/10.1016/j.fertnstert.2021.02.019.
45. Hill MA. The stain of slavery on the black women's body and the development gynecology: historical trauma of a black women's body. Macksey J. 2020;1:1.
46. Grundstrom H, Engman L, Rimhagen E, Soderstierna C, Flink I. Experiences of communication in women with endometriosis: perceived validation and invalidation in different contexts, and associations with health-related quality of life. J Psychosom Obstet Gynaecol. 2023;44(1):2264483. https://doi.org/10.1080/0167482X.2023.2264483.
47. Slade P, O'Neill C, Simpson AJ, Lashen H. The relationship between perceived stigma, disclosure patterns, support and distress in new attendees at an infertility clinic. Hum Reprod. 2007;22(8):2309–17. https://doi.org/10.1093/humrep/dem115.
48. Lawson AK. Caution is warranted when discussing correlations between stress and reproductive outcomes. Fertil Steril. 2020;114(5):972–3. https://doi.org/10.1016/j.fertnstert.2020.07.054.
49. Weathers FW, Litz BT, Keane TM, Palmieri PA, Marx BP, Schnurr PP (2013b) The PTSD checklist for DSM-5 (PCL-5). Retrieved from www.ptsd.va.gov
50. Prins A, Bovin MJ, Kimerling R, Kaloupek DG, Marx BP, Pless Kaiser A, Schnurr PP (2015) Primary care PTSD screen for DSM-5 (PC-PTSD-5). Retrieved from https://www.ptsd.va.gov
51. Weathers FW, Blake DD, Schnurr PP, Kaloupek DG, Marx BP, Keane TM (2013a) The life events checklist for DSM-5 (LEC-5). Retrieved from www.ptsd.va.gov

Chapter 2
Trauma-Informed Care in the Setting of Pregnancy Loss

Chloe Warlick and Susan C. Klock

Introduction

Pregnancy loss is relatively common and affects between 15% and 25% of all pregnancies. It increases with maternal age with rates between 9% and 12% in women under 35 years of age and up to 50% in women over 40 years old [1]. The most common types of pregnancy losses are early losses which are often defined as clinical pregnancies (i.e., visualized on ultrasound) which result in miscarriage prior to 20 weeks of gestation. Although biochemical pregnancy losses and ectopic pregnancies are not considered clinical pregnancies and thus not always recognized as a pregnancy loss by healthcare professionals, biochemical pregnancy losses are the most common type of loss and both experiences are often considered pregnancy losses by the patients who experience them [2, 3]. Although not traditionally considered a reproductive loss in the medical world, some patients also view failed embryo transfers and destruction of supernumerary embryos as a deep emotional loss of a potential child [4]. Although most pregnancy loss research focuses on people assigned female at birth, it is important to recognize that not all pregnancies are carried by people that identify as women. Moving forward, we use the term women because the research we discuss was conducted on women.

Within the broad domain of pregnancy loss there is a unique subset of women who experience recurrent pregnancy loss. The American Society for Reproductive

C. Warlick
Department of Psychiatry and Behavioral Sciences, Northwestern University Feinberg School of Medicine, Chicago, IL, USA
e-mail: chloe.warlick@northwestern.edu

S. C. Klock (✉)
Departments of Obstetrics and Gynecology & Psychiatry, Northwestern University Feinberg School of Medicine, Chicago, IL, USA
e-mail: sck318@northwestern.edu

A. K. Lawson, A. Swanson (eds.), *Trauma-Informed Reproductive Healthcare*,
https://doi.org/10.1007/978-3-031-67474-7_2

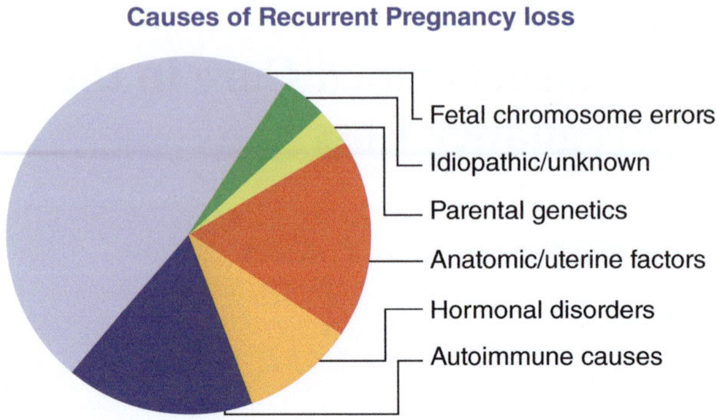

Fig. 2.1 Estimated causes of recurrent pregnancy loss

Medicine (ASRM) Practice committee defines recurrent pregnancy loss as the loss of two or more clinical pregnancies documented by ultrasound. ASRM also delineates recurrent pregnancy loss (RPL) as a disease distinct from infertility which affects between 1% and 3% of reproductive aged women [5]. Primary RPL refers to multiple pregnancy losses in a woman who does not have a previous live birth and secondary RPL refers to repeated losses in a woman who has had a previous pregnancy.

There are many potential causes for RPL [6, 7] including genetics, age, abnormal uterine anatomy, chronic endometritis, antiphospholipid syndrome, inherited thrombophilias, and sperm quality (Fig. 2.1). In approximately 50% of cases, a presumptive diagnosis will be made; in the other 50% no causative factor will be identified. In cases of unexplained RPL, women often presume that psychological or lifestyle stress may play a causative role, although direct evidence for a causal role of psychological stress in the etiology of RPL is lacking. Many women with RPL will go on to have healthy, ongoing pregnancies, in fact, women with RPL have a high likelihood of having a baby. According to data by Lund et al. [8] women with at least three previous pregnancy losses had a 66–80% chance of subsequent live birth within 5 years of the first consultation at a specialty RPL clinic (Fig. 2.2). However, experiencing RPL can have a significant psychological impact on the woman and her partner. Bailey et al. [9] have noted, "recurrent miscarriage represents an extremely distressing condition that can be both physically and emotionally traumatizing." The physical aspects of the loss; pain, bleeding, possible surgical intervention in an emergent setting are remembered long after the pregnancy is lost. The feelings surrounding the loss and the psychological reverberations can prompt fears of another loss, the loss of the wished for child, fear of never becoming a parent, and anticipatory anxiety about future pregnancies.

Pregnancy losses that occur in the later perinatal time frame are equally if not more psychologically distressing than both early and recurrent pregnancy loss. For example, losses occurring after 24 weeks (e.g., stillbirths) are often psychologically and physically traumatic [10]. Termination for medical reasons similarly often happen in the second trimester as a result of medical conditions identified at a 20-week pregnancy ultrasound. Although it is the intended parents' decision to terminate the

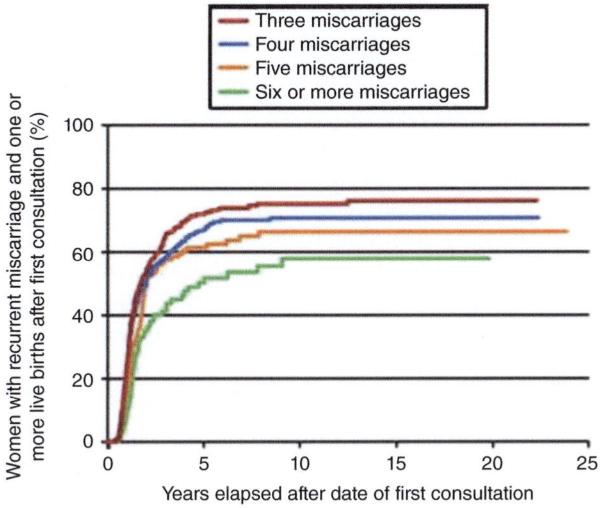

Fig. 2.2 Chances of successful pregnancy after recurrent pregnancy loss (from Lund et al, used with permission)

pregnancy, the pregnancy is often a highly desired one and the termination is experienced as a pregnancy loss albeit with stigma likely being associated with their decision and thus decreased sharing and/or support from loved ones [11].

Review of the Literature

Early Pregnancy Loss

Pregnancy loss, regardless of when it occurs, can have a profound psychological impact on the person who experiences it, their partner, and others in their support network. Research indicates that even early pregnancy losses can lead to psychological distress, including depression, anxiety, and trauma-related disorders. For example, Farren and colleagues (2016) investigated emotional distress in women following early pregnancy loss (EPL), defined as a loss before 20 weeks gestation (including ectopic pregnancy), compared to a control group with ongoing pregnancies. One month after pregnancy loss, the EPL group exhibited higher psychological morbidity, with 28% meeting criteria for probable PTSD, 32% for anxiety, and 16% for depression. Interestingly, whether the loss was due to ectopic pregnancy or miscarriage did not significantly affect distress levels. The control group reported lower rates of anxiety and depression (10%), with no cases of probable PTSD. Three months post-pregnancy loss, probable PTSD symptoms persisted and increased to 38%, while anxiety and depression rates decreased to 20% and 5%, respectively [12].

The partners of those who experience early pregnancy loss also report distress following these losses. Although most research on pregnancy loss focuses on the emotional experiences of cisgender heterosexual women following pregnancy loss, comparative examinations of their male partners' emotional experiences suggest that men also experience grief and symptoms of traumatic stress. However, men may be less likely to share their internal emotional experiences of grief with others, particularly their partners thus reducing the recognition and support of their grief [13, 14]. Similarly, female partners in lesbian couples and gay men using fertility treatments to grow their families experience symptoms of grief, anxiety, and depression but may also not receive adequate emotional support during or following pregnancy loss [15–17]. Finally, gestational carriers may also experience symptoms of grief and traumatic stress following losses [18].

Society's tendency to dismiss perinatal loss as legitimate grief for the pregnant person, their partner or for those growing their families via gestational surrogacy can make it challenging for bereaved parents to openly express their emotions. This can lead to disenfranchised grief (i.e., grief that is not recognized by others as valid), which may evolve into traumatic grief, especially for those who experience early pregnancy loss [19]. Lack of social support and limited opportunities to share grief experiences related to pregnancy loss exacerbate emotional distress for all parties no matter when in the gestational period the loss occurs [20].

Recurrent Pregnancy Loss

It is well documented that RPL results in significant psychological distress including anxiety, depression, and self-blame. Kolte et al. [21] explored the psychological impact of RPL in a cross-sectional study of 301 women with RPL (≥3 losses) and compared them to a group of women who were trying to conceive. 8.6% of the women in the RPL group had depression scores consistent with moderate to severe depression, compared to 2.2% of the women in the comparison group. Women in the RPL group also had significantly higher self-reported stress scores than the comparison group. Other studies of women and their male partners have found the risk of emotional distress for those experiencing RPL to be as high as: 51.7% for women and 19.1% for their male partners for depression; 47.7% for women and 19.1% of men for clinical anxiety; 28.6% of RPL women and 10.7% for their male partners for high stress; 13.7% of women and 3.9% of men for PTSD diagnosis (with women reporting significantly higher scores than men on subscales assessing intrusion and hyperarousal); and with 28.1% of women and 30.7% of men receiving limited social support [22–24]. It should be noted that although men's distress levels are generally found to be lower than that of RPL women, it has been posited that the lower level of distress in male partners may be due to their feeling that they have to remain positive and hopeful which influenced responding; alternatively, the male partners may have had difficulty identifying and naming their emotions; or that results were due to the differential impact of the physiological experience of the pregnancy loss (i.e., women experience greater levels of depression and stress because of the physical experience of the loss and the fluctuations of reproductive hormones during and after the pregnancy loss) [22].

The experience of anxiety, and in particular symptoms of PTSD, are evident in the strategies women with RPL use to cope with subsequent pregnancies. For example, Bailey et al. [9] conducted a qualitative study of 14 women with RPL to describe how these women experience a new pregnancy in the setting of their RPL history. The analysis elucidated several organizing or overarching themes which describe the RPL woman's experience. Those themes were: (1) turmoil of emotion; (2) preparing for the worst; (3) setting of personal milestones; (4) hypervigilance (5) social isolation; (6) adoption of a pragmatic approach and; (7) need for professional affirmation. The first theme, turmoil of emotion represented the woman's reported feeling of many emotions at the beginning of a new pregnancy is consistent with Criterion B symptoms of PTSD (i.e., cognitively intrusive experiences that cause distress). They reported feeling excited, yet worried about the future of the pregnancy and ruminating over the future of the pregnancy and feeling uncertain of its outcome. All the participants reported significant levels of anxiety and worry that felt overwhelming and interfered with other areas of their lives. Patients also reported guilt over prior pregnancy losses and letting down their partner or family. Women also noted shame at feeling jealous or envious of other pregnant women. These negative alterations in thoughts are consistent with symptoms of Criterion D of PTSD.

The second theme, preparing for the worst, represented the emotional and cognitive strategies women used to keep themselves grounded and not get too excited or hopeful about the new pregnancy. This is consistent with Criterion C of PTSD (i.e., avoidance of distressing psychological and physical stimuli) and included thoughts of suppressing hope about the pregnancy and not thinking into the future in reference to the pregnancy. A third theme that women reported was that of setting and meeting milestones within the pregnancy. The women described breaking the pregnancy down into smaller time frames (days, weeks) to navigate their progress through the first trimester and to continue to progress past previous gestation durations or making it to new obstetric visit milestones. This third theme may also consistent with Criterion C of PTSD as appears to involve avoidance of thoughts of the pregnancy at a future stage. The hypervigilance theme (an example of the Criterion E symptoms for PTSD) was illustrated by close monitoring of symptoms of early pregnancy such as nausea, tiredness, or breast tenderness as evidence of the ongoing nature of the pregnancy. Frequently seeking reassurance from healthcare professionals that their pregnancy was ongoing was a common manifestation of this theme. Another example of avoidance behaviors associated with Criterion C of PTSD; social isolation was the fifth theme identified in the study. This theme referred to women's common pattern of not sharing the news of another pregnancy with others and limiting their social interactions with others while waiting for the early weeks of pregnancy to pass. Often women feared that the current pregnancy would result in a miscarriage therefore there was no need to tell others of the pregnancy. Women also noted adopting a pragmatic approach to manage the anxiety related to the pregnancy. They reported using distraction techniques and keeping busy to make time feel as if it was passing more quickly. Work often provided a needed distraction during early pregnancy. Women also reported engaging in lifestyle behavior changes that they thought may reduce the risk of another miscarriage. The last organizing theme that emerged from the interview data was the need for professional affirmation. This refers to women's wish for more frequent contact with their healthcare professionals during the early waiting period of a new pregnancy. Also, they wanted more acknowledgment of the fears and anxieties associated with a new pregnancy in the setting of RPL. The results of Bailey's study highlight that the waiting time in a new pregnancy among women who have experienced RPL is often difficult and traumatic.

Taken together, based on the review of the studies presented here, it is clear that a subset of women and men who experience RPL may also suffer from symptoms of PTSD with some exhibiting a subset of such symptoms and some meeting full diagnostic criteria for the disorder. They have direct exposure to a significant stressor (PTSD Criterion A), the pregnancy loss. They have persistent intrusive thoughts and emotional distress after exposures to reminders of the loss (PTSD Criterion B). In addition, they may engage in avoidant coping behaviors (e.g., avoiding pregnant people and babies/children) as they navigate interacting with others (PTSD Criterion C). They experience negative alterations in thoughts and mood by developing an overly pessimistic outlook on the viability of future pregnancies (PTSD Criterion D) and often engage in hypervigilant behaviors once they are pregnant again (PTSD Criterion E). As with other vulnerable populations, it is important to screen women with pregnancy loss and their partners for symptoms related to PTSD, depression, and anxiety.

If clinically significant symptoms are present, provision of specialized psychological care for women and their partners is an important part of the management plan. As Dimitriadis [7] noted, psychological support "should be patient-centered, provided in a clinic dedicated to early pregnancy loss, include the partner and acknowledge that miscarriage is a momentous life event." However, there have been few studies of the provision of psychological interventions for women with RPL. Older studies looking at the provision of psychological intervention for women who had experienced RPL were grounded in the belief that psychological stress played a causative role in RPL thereby blaming women for causing their own reproductive losses. Although these studies showed a positive effect of psychological intervention by comparing the provision of specialized psychological support to standard care, these studies were limited by small sample size, lack of randomized assignment to the intervention group, problematic study design with failure to control for relevant variables, and other concerns [25–27].

More recently, Jensen et al. [28] conducted a nonblinded RCT of a 7-week meditation and mindfulness intervention to reduce stress among women referred to a specialty RPL clinic. Women with high prescreening levels of stress and no symptoms of clinical depression were invited to participate in the study. The researchers compared the impact of the 7-week intervention on levels of perceived stress, fertility problem stress, and marital benefit among 38 women with RPL in the intervention group compared to 38 women in the routine care group. The authors found that perceived stressed significantly decreased in both the intervention and control group, but the intervention group had a significantly larger decrease in stress and this decrease in perceived stress was still evident at the 12-month follow-up assessment. Of note, the reproductive outcomes at 12 months were not significantly different between the two groups.

Late Pregnancy Losses

The psychological impact of pregnancy loss is not limited to early gestation or recurrent pregnancy loss. Later-stage losses, such as stillbirths and terminations for medical reasons, can be immensely psychologically distressing. Research shows that these losses can profoundly affect individuals, leading to intense grief, feelings of emptiness, and a deep sense of loss [29]. Social and cultural factors, such as stigma, can further compound these psychological challenges for those who experience stillbirth or a medical pregnancy termination [30, 31].

It is not uncommon for those who experience a late pregnancy loss to develop symptoms of PTSD. A 2021 systematic review by Westby and colleagues [31] summarized findings from 13 empirical studies on parents' psychological outcomes after experiencing stillbirth, defined as fetal death at or after 20 weeks of gestation. The review indicated that stillbirth is associated with symptoms of depression, anxiety, and PTSD, which are most severe immediately after the loss but tend to decrease over time. However, some individuals may develop chronic psychological symptoms. Risk factors for distress include younger age, lower income, and no prior pregnancies, while strong social support serves as a protective factor. Being unmarried was associated with a higher risk of depression, and high perceived social support reduced re-experiencing symptoms of PTSD at 3 and 6 months post-stillbirth.

Terminating a pregnancy due to fetal anomaly (TOPFA) is another stigmatized form of pregnancy loss associated with complicated grief, trauma, and depression. The process of undergoing a TOPFA engenders various opportunities for experiencing psychological distress, including the diagnosis of the fetal anomaly, the decision to undergo a TOPFA, the time between the decision and the procedure, the TOPFA itself, and the recovery post-termination, all of which are independently distressing and potentially traumatizing [32]. Hanschmidt and colleagues (2018) conducted a study with 148 women who experienced TOPFA in Germany, with most terminations occurring in the second trimester. They found that perceived stigma at the time of the termination was associated with greater levels of depression, posttraumatic stress, anxiety, and complicated grief. Internalized stigma was linked to the persistence of these symptoms in the long term [32]. Recent changes in law in the USA, specifically Dobbs vs. Jackson Women's Health Organization in 2022 and many state laws, have significantly limited access to care for TOPFA. This change has made the access of care difficult for patients such that they may need to travel out of state to a medical system that they are unfamiliar with in order to access TOPFA. Additionally, this change in law may also increase the social stigma for accessing TOPFA.

In light of the research showing increased risk of psychological distress including PTSD for those experiencing late-term pregnancy losses, it is crucial for women facing long-lasting psychological difficulties following TOPFA or stillbirth to receive interventions addressing internalized stigma, such as guilt, shame, or self-blame. These studies underscore the need for healthcare professionals to combat the stigma surrounding late-term pregnancy losses and adopt a trauma-informed approach to mitigate psychological distress in affected individuals. More research is needed into the type and format of psychological interventions for women and their partners who experience pregnancy loss. When providing psychological interventions to this patient population, the tenets of trauma-informed care can provide a useful framework.

Trauma-Informed Care During/Following Pregnancy Loss

Multidisciplinary care by physicians, mental health professionals, nurses, and other medical professionals who are well versed in pregnancy loss is a first step in creating a safe and secure treatment environment for patients. Acknowledging and validating the psychological impact of all types of pregnancy losses and offering routine psychological support services that are integrated into medical care can normalize and validate the psychosocial impact of the patient's experience. Discussing the treatment modality, frequency and timing of visits, and engaging the patient in determining the support that best fits for them can enhance feelings of choice and control. Professional, empathic, evidence-based care can build the foundation of trustworthiness and strong therapeutic alliance. As psychological support is provided, the goal of patient empowerment can be reached by helping the patient find ways to process their thoughts and feelings about RPL, explore the meaning of their experience, identify areas of efficacy, restore their reproductive self-esteem and ultimately help them meet their family building goals.

The experience of perinatal loss can be uniquely and profoundly distressing for those it affects, and healthcare professionals hold a pivotal role in alleviating trauma and facilitating the healing process. Research underscores the beneficial influence of trauma-informed healthcare for those experiencing reproductive losses. For instance, research shows that intended parents who received compassionate emotional support from healthcare professionals upon receiving a pregnancy loss diagnosis reported significantly lower levels of grief after the loss of their child [20] and clinicians who exhibited non-judgmental kindness and tender care toward their patients and their babies were perceived as the most reassuring and comforting figures during the emotionally taxing experience of pregnancy loss [11].

A framework of care based on the Substance Abuse and Mental Health Services Administration (SAMHSA) model of trauma-informed care has been developed specifically for those experiencing pregnancy loss. This model is guided by the belief that pregnancy loss patients should be "companioned rather than treated"

([19], p. 918) and encompasses the six core trauma-informed care principles: safety, trustworthiness, peer support, collaboration, empowerment, choice, and consideration of cultural, historical, and gender issues and can be utilized for patients experiencing reproductive losses at any gestational age [19]. Berry applied this framework to minimize traumatic impact on those experiencing pregnancy loss which include the time at which the patient learns of the loss, at the time of a stillbirth, when communicating the experience of loss to others, and after physical completion of the loss [19].

To promote healing and reduce the traumatic impact of the initial phase wherein the patient learns about the loss and/or fetal diagnosis, trauma-informed healthcare professionals can apply the following strategies:

- Create a serene and distraction-free environment when sharing the news of the loss or fetal diagnosis.
- Use clear and empathetic communication, avoiding medical jargon and terms like "non-viable" and avoidance of false hope.
- Recognize that patients may perceive failed embryo transfers, biochemical pregnancy losses, ectopic pregnancies, and supernumerary embryo dispositions as pregnancy losses and provide emotional validation for these losses.
- Ensure the patient comprehends the information and emphasize their involvement in decision-making.
- Allocate ample time for addressing questions and helping the patient process the information.

In cases of stillbirth, trauma-informed healthcare professionals should consider the following suggestions in order to reduce harm and promote healing:

- Remaining present during the birthing process, demonstrating attentiveness to the patient's needs, remaining flexible, and avoiding attempts to "fix" the patient's emotional pain.
- Suggesting meaningful experiences based on the patient's preferences without pressure, such as giving the baby a bath, taking photographs, holding the baby, or involving siblings.
- Allowing the patient to dictate their level of participation in the birthing process.
- Offer the option for patients to leave through a separate exit to avoid encounters with celebrating families.

Disclosing the loss to others in the patients' social network can be particularly traumatizing given the need to discuss the trauma as well as hurtful comments or questions by those hearing about the loss. Thus, to assist patients in disclosing the loss to others, trauma-informed healthcare professionals should consider:

- Preparing patients for potential insensitive comments from well-meaning individuals.
- Providing information on the importance of social support during challenging times and discussing available resources.
- Validating the patient's feelings of grief.

Lastly, for follow-up care after the loss, the framework can be implemented in the following ways:

- Maintain follow-up care for at least 1 year after the loss.
- Sustain communication with patients to offer ongoing support.
- Provide education, resources, and support on various topics like lactation, parenting living children, grief, and partner intimacy.
- Reach out to patients on significant dates with cards, phone calls, or text messages to offer continued support and care.

In fostering a supportive and healing environment for parents navigating perinatal loss, a comprehensive approach that encompasses both the physical and non-physical facets of care is imperative. This entails the provision of dedicated spaces designed to minimize potential triggers for grieving parents; effective and collaborative communication among healthcare team members (including mental health professionals, chaplains, and child life specialists); emotionally validating communication with the patient, partner, and support people; and continued care after the loss. Furthermore, prioritizing the well-being of staff is essential, as repeated exposure to sharing bad news and/or witnessing patient trauma can be traumatizing. Training programs aimed at mitigating vicarious trauma, which is a known factor contributing to burnout and reduced job satisfaction are therefore vital for those working with patients at risk of reproductive loss.

Conclusions

Early pregnancy losses, recurrent pregnancy losses, and late-term losses are often profoundly emotionally distressing to patients and their partners. Like trauma, loss is in the eye of the beholder and patients often consider non-clinically recognized reproductive losses (e.g., biochemical pregnancy loss, ectopic pregnancy, failed embryo transfer) as intensely painful pregnancy losses. The failure to appropriately validate and emotionally support individuals during and after pregnancy loss increases the risk of psychological distress. Pregnancy loss is a physically and psychologically stressful experience and a subset of women and men may develop PTSD or PTSD symptoms. Specialized trauma-informed medical and psychological care for these patients is an important part of a multidisciplinary approach to care.

References

1. El Hachem H, Crepaux V, May-Panloup P, Descamps P, Legendre G, Bouet PE. Recurrent pregnancy loss: current perspectives. Int J Women's Health. 2017;9:331–45.
2. Macklon NS, Geraedts JP, Fauser BC. Conception to ongoing pregnancy: the 'black box' of early pregnancy loss. Hum Reprod Update. 2002;8(4):333–43.

3. Purandare N, Ryan G, Ciprike V, Trevisan J, Sheehan J, Geary M. Grieving after early pregnancy loss—a common reality. Ir Med J. 2012;105(10):326–8.
4. de Lacey S. Death in the clinic: women's perceptions and experiences of discarding supernumerary IVF embryos. Sociol Health Illn. 2017;39(3):397–411.
5. The Practice Committee of the American Society for Reproductive Medicine. Evaluation and treatment of RPL: a committee opinion. Fertil Steril. 2012;98:1103–11.
6. Ford HB, Schust DJ. Recurrent pregnancy loss: etiology, diagnosis, and therapy. Rev Obstet Gynecol. 2009;2(2):76–83.
7. Dimitriadis E, Menkhorst E, Saito S, Kutteh WH, Brosens JJ. Recurrent pregnancy loss. Nat Rev Dis Primers. 2020;6(1):98.
8. Lund M, Kamper-Jorgensen M, Nielsen HS, Lidegaard O, Andersen AM, Christiansen OB. Prognosis for live birth in women with recurrent miscarriage: what is the best measure of success? Obstet Gynecol. 2012;119(1):37–43.
9. Bailey SL, Boivin J, Cheong YC, Kitson-Reynolds E, Bailey C, Macklon N. Hope for the best ...but expect the worst: a qualitative study to explore how women with recurrent miscarriage experience the early waiting period of a new pregnancy. BMJ Open. 2019;9(5):e029354.
10. Horsch A, Jacobs I, McKenzie-McHarg K. Cognitive predictors and risk factors of PTSD following stillbirth: a short-term longitudinal study. J Trauma Stress. 2015;28(2):110–7.
11. Heaney S, Tomlinson M, Aventin A. Termination of pregnancy for fetal anomaly: a systematic review of the healthcare experiences and needs of parents. BMC Pregnancy Childbirth. 2022;22(1):441.
12. Farren J, Jalmbrant M, Ameye L, Joash K, Mitchell-Jones N, Tapp S, et al. Post-traumatic stress, anxiety and depression following miscarriage or ectopic pregnancy: a prospective cohort study. BMJ Open. 2016;6(11):e011864.
13. Obst KL, Due C. Australian men's experiences of support following pregnancy loss: a qualitative study. Midwifery. 2019;70:1–6.
14. Farren J, Jalmbrant M, Falconieri N, Mitchell-Jones N, Bobdiwala S, Al-Memar M, et al. Differences in post-traumatic stress, anxiety and depression following miscarriage or ectopic pregnancy between women and their partners: multicenter prospective cohort study. Ultrasound Obstet Gynecol. 2021;57(1):141–8.
15. Riggs DW, Due C, Power J. Gay men's experiences of surrogacy clinics in India. J Fam Plann Reprod Health Care. 2015;41(1):48–53.
16. Wojnar D. Miscarriage experiences of lesbian couples. J Midwifery Womens Health. 2007;52(5):479–85.
17. Peel E. Pregnancy loss in lesbian and bisexual women: an online survey of experiences. Hum Reprod. 2010;25(3):721–7.
18. Berend Z. Surrogate losses: understandings of pregnancy loss and assisted reproduction among surrogate mothers. Med Anthropol Q. 2010;24(2):240–62.
19. Berry SN, Winsor T, Huene L. A proposed framework for perinatal loss trauma informed care. J Neonatal Nurs. 2023;29(6):916–21.
20. Berry S. The trauma of perinatal loss: a scoping review. Trauma Care. 2022;2(3):392–407.
21. Kolte AM, Olsen LR, Mikkelsen EM, Christiansen OB, Nielsen HS. Depression and emotional stress is highly prevalent among women with recurrent pregnancy loss. Hum Reprod. 2015;30(4):777–82.
22. Hedegaard S, Landersoe SK, Olsen LR, Krog MC, Kolte AM, Nielsen HS. Stress and depression among women and men who have experienced recurrent pregnancy loss: focusing on both sexes. Reprod Biomed Online. 2021;42(6):1172–80.
23. Voss P, Schick M, Langer L, Ainsworth A, Ditzen B, Strowitzki T, et al. Recurrent pregnancy loss: a shared stressor—couple-orientated psychological research findings. Fertil Steril. 2020;114(6):1288–96.
24. Kuhlmann E, Scharli P, Schick M, Ditzen B, Langer L, Strowitzki T, et al. The posttraumatic impact of recurrent pregnancy loss in both women and men. Geburtshilfe Frauenheilkd. 2023;83(1):88–96.

25. Stray-Pedersen B, Stray-Pedersen S. Etiologic factors and subsequent reproductive performance in 195 couples with a prior history of habitual abortion. Am J Obstet Gynecol. 1984;148(2):140–6.
26. Nakano Y, Akechi T, Furukawa TA, Sugiura-Ogasawara M. Cognitive behavior therapy for psychological distress in patients with recurrent miscarriage. Psychol Res Behav Manag. 2013;6:37–43.
27. Stray-Pedersen B, Stray-Pedersen S. Recurrent abortion: the role of psychotherapy. In: Beard RW, Ship F, editors. Early pregnancy loss: mechanisms and treatment. New York: NY: Springer-Verlag; 1988. p. 433–40.
28. Jensen KHK, Krog MC, Koert E, Hedegaard S, Chonovitsch M, Schmidt L, et al. Meditation and mindfulness reduce perceived stress in women with recurrent pregnancy loss: a randomized controlled trial. Reprod Biomed Online. 2021;43(2):246–56.
29. Quenby S, Gallos ID, Dhillon-Smith RK, Podesek M, Stephenson MD, Fisher J, et al. Miscarriage matters: the epidemiological, physical, psychological, and economic costs of early pregnancy loss. Lancet. 2021;397(10285):1658–67.
30. Hendrix T, Roncoroni J, Magdamo B, Whitaker S, Zareba K, Grieco N. Stigma, social support, and decision satisfaction in terminations of pregnancy for medical reasons. Womens Health Rep (New Rochelle). 2023;4(1):271–9.
31. Westby CL, Erlandsen AR, Nilsen SA, Visted E, Thimm JC. Depression, anxiety, PTSD, and OCD after stillbirth: a systematic review. BMC Pregnancy Childbirth. 2021;21(1):782.
32. Hanschmidt F, Treml J, Klingner J, Stepan H, Kersting A. Stigma in the context of pregnancy termination after diagnosis of fetal anomaly: associations with grief, trauma, and depression. Arch Womens Ment Health. 2018;21(4):391–9.

Chapter 3
Trauma-Informed Care in Patients with a History of Sexual Trauma

Aisha Kazi and Angela Lawson

Introduction

As has been made clear in other chapters in this book, the provision of trauma-informed health care is vital for individuals who have experienced one or more traumatic events. Those who have experienced trauma(s) often experience a loss of power and control during the traumatic event(s) and trauma-informed health care empowers patients to be more involved in decisions related to and control of their health care. Trauma-informed health care also recognizes the ways in which trauma is manifested in all aspects of the individual's life and actively seeks to avoid retraumatizing patients by reducing these triggers and providing compassionate stigma-free care. Overall, trauma-informed care aids in the development of trust between health care professionals (HCP) and patients and can be considered a component of patient-centered care [1].

Sexual victimization, which includes sexual assault or harassment and other unwanted experiences (e.g., non-consensual taking or distribution of images of a sexual nature), is unfortunately highly prevalent in the USA and internationally. Sexual assault and attempted sexual assault describe a situation in which an assailant forces (or attempts to force) an individual to participate in various sexual acts, often but not always including penetration. Sexual harassment can occur in many environments but is often discussed within the context of harassment in the workplace or schools and may be perpetrated by those with power over the victim (e.g., professors, supervisors, someone in a position of authority/seniority), by colleagues/co-workers, or others with whom the employee interacts at work or school. Sexual

A. Kazi
Chicago, IL, USA

A. Lawson (✉)
Obstetrics and Gynecology, Northwestern Medicine, Chicago, IL, USA
e-mail: alawsonphd@gmail.com

A. Lawson, A. Swanson (eds.), *Trauma-Informed Reproductive Healthcare*,
https://doi.org/10.1007/978-3-031-67474-7_3

harassment includes "unwelcome sexual advances, requests for sexual favors, and other verbal or physical conduct of a sexual nature" if (1) such behaviors interfere with the person's work or otherwise create a hostile work environment or (2) if such behaviors affect employment related decisions such as promotion or termination [2].

Although numerous published rates of sexual assault and harassment exist, they are underestimates given that few survivors of sexual assault and/or sexual harassment formally report their experiences due to concerns related to how they will be treated (e.g., stigmatized) upon disclosure [3]. However, estimates of the prevalence of sexual assault in the USA from the National Violence Against Women Survey (NVAWS) and the National Intimate Partner and Sexual Violence Survey (NISVS) suggest that at least 20% of American women have been sexually assaulted [4, 5]. The World Health Organization (WHO) similarly estimates that as many as 30% of women worldwide have experienced sexual and/or other interpersonal violence [6]. Although this will be discussed in further detail in other chapters, it should be noted that certain individuals are at greater risk of sexual victimization than others. These include LGBTQ+ individuals, children, those belonging to certain racial/ethnic groups, those who are disabled, and those who are incarcerated [5, 7–9]. Research examining all types of sexual victimization indicate that unwanted sexual touching and sexual harassment are likely even more commonly experienced by women than is rape with studies showing 40–75% of women and 13–31% of men in the USA having reported experiencing workplace sexual harassment and >40% of women and nearly 25% of men having experienced any kind of unwanted sexual contact violence in their lifetimes [10–14]. The majority of those who experience sexual victimization are assaulted or harassed by someone with whom they are acquainted (e.g., social acquaintance, intimate partner, coworker, supervisor) and research on sexual victimization often finds women to be the more common survivor of sexual assault and harassment with men being most likely to perpetrate such acts [2, 5].

It is well known that sexual assault and sexual harassment may lead to the survivor developing symptoms consistent with a diagnosis of Posttraumatic Stress Disorder (PTSD), Major Depressive Disorder, Eating Disorders, Panic Disorder, and/or other symptoms of psychological distress or disorder. For example, a recent meta-analysis of 22 studies ($N = 2106$) of sexual assault survivors reported that the majority of survivors experience symptoms of PTSD immediately following the assault with nearly 75% of survivors meeting diagnostic criteria for PTSD within a month of being assaulted and nearly 50% continuing to experience these symptoms a year after the assault occurred [15].

In addition to psychological distress and disorder, sexual victimization has also been shown to be associated with childhood and teenage academic achievement (e.g., lower grade point average, learning difficulties, and dropping out of college), negative health outcomes and behaviors (e.g., chronic pelvic pain, gastrointestinal problems, sexual dysfunction, pain disorders, obesity, substance use, smoking, risky sex behaviors, decreased engagement in exercise, injury, sexually transmitted illnesses, unintended pregnancy, etc.), occupational/economic difficulties, relationship/intimacy problems, and other negative outcomes [5, 16–21].

Workplace sexual harassment has similarly been associated with a host of negative outcomes. A seminal study on the antecedents and consequences of workplace harassment found that women who experienced such behaviors reported experiencing psychological distress such as PTSD symptoms, decreased health satisfaction, absenteeism, and intention to leave their jobs more than those who were not harassed [22]. A subsequent meta-analysis which included 44 studies (N = 68,343 women and men) confirmed that sexual harassment was associated with decreased job satisfaction, organizational commitment, work productivity, and PTSD symptomatology [12]. Additional research on psychological outcomes of sexual harassment found that the majority of women (N = 1218) women who participated in a class action lawsuit alleging workplace harassment at a large national financial services organization reported experiencing symptoms of PTSD, depression, decreased health and life satisfaction, and eating disorder symptoms as a result of the harassing experience and these symptoms persisted even after the lawsuit was resolved. Additionally, women who did not participate in the class action (N = 465) but also worked at the same organization, reported experiencing symptoms of PTSD and eating disorder symptoms which also developed as a result of their alleged experience(s) of being harassed at the organization [23].

Even in the absence of full diagnostic criteria for PTSD, Major Depressive Disorder or other psychological condition, survivors of sexual assault, sexual harassment and/or other sexual victimization must navigate a world post-victimization that is rife with stimuli (i.e., triggers) which remind them of the assault or harassment. Many who experience sexual victimization are distressed when exposed to such noxious stimuli and actively avoid situations, people, thoughts/feelings, and/or people which remind them of the distressing experience. Indeed avoidance-based reactions to trauma stimuli and the distressing reactions to such stimuli reflect two criteria for a diagnosis of PTSD in the Diagnostic and Statistical Manual of Mental Disorders-fifth edition (DSM-5) [24]. Efforts to avoid exposure to trauma stimuli and/or negative reactions by trusted individuals may lead survivors to not disclose their experiences to family, those in their social networks, and even their healthcare professionals. Desire to avoid distress may also lead patients to avoid healthcare (e.g., pelvic/breast exams, semen analysis, colonoscopy, psychotherapy) which exposes them to trauma stimuli such as physical touching or discussion of the traumatic event or its sequelae [25]. Patients with a history of sexual victimization who engage in such personal and invasive medical exams may experience an exacerbation of their trauma-related symptoms of depression and/or anxiety as they are reminded of the loss of sense of control and power they experienced during their prior traumatic experience(s) [26].

Despite the well-established risk of serious physical and psychological consequences following sexual victimization, research shows that it is uncommon for medical professionals to ask patients about either childhood or later experiences of sexual victimization. For example, Farrow et al. found than among 145 physician members of the American College of Obstetricians and Gynecologist only 29% reported screening for childhood sexual abuse at least "most of the time" and only 23.4% similarly reported screening for PTSD symptoms. Barriers to screening included lack of time, training, and mental health resources necessary to effectively screen. [25]. Patients may not voluntarily disclose their experience of sexual victimization to their HCPs, but this does not mean that they do not want their HCPs to ask them about their histories of abuse. Indeed, numerous studies show that the majority of female patients who have experienced sexual victimization want their physicians to ask them about such experiences [25, 27, 28]. Additionally, although the #MeToo movement helped raise awareness of the frequency and psychological consequences of sexual victimization, little to no research has been conducted which assesses the screening of such experiences by HCPs among male patient populations. Given the greater awareness of and yet low screening for sexual assault in female patients as compared to male patients, it is likely that the experience of sexual harassment of both women and men remains rarely assessed within heath care settings. It is also important to remember that although many perpetrators of sexual abuse are men, women have also been found to commit such violence; HCPs should not assume that any patient is immune from the risk of sexual victimization by either a male or female perpetrator.

Screening for a history of sexual victimization among patients seeking healthcare is needed in order to appropriately counsel and/or reduce patient risk of negative health outcomes (e.g., avoidance of seeking health care) as well as to provide a safe and supportive environment for survivors to receive care [29]. For example, counseling a patient about the medical need to reduce substance use which fails to take into consideration that the patient is using those substances (albeit maladaptively) as a means to "self-medicate" and sooth their trauma-related anxious or depressive symptoms (which are unknown to the HCP) would likely be ineffective in reducing substance use as the healthcare professional is not able to discuss a realistic alternative coping method. However, even if such screening does not occur, it appears likely that the provision of trauma-informed care to all patients may lead to increased patient comfort with disclosure of traumatic experiences. For example, one study of $N = 143$ female patients found that patients were more likely to disclose their history of sexual victimization if their HCP provided a safe and supportive environment in which the healthcare professional had a positive attitude, was not judgmental, was not rushed, provided a comfortable environment, and was trusted by the patient [28]. Numerous other studies similarly find that a safe, supportive, and non-judgmental environment increases the likelihood of disclosure [29].

Although it appears that many HCPs believe that it is important and part of their responsibility to screen for a history of sexual victimization and are unlikely to reliably guess who has a history of trauma, it appears unlikely that routine screening will be a reality in every health care setting due to various barriers in screening [25]. Given that it is well known that most people will experience at least one traumatic experience in their life whether during childhood or adulthood and that most women and many men will experience sexual victimization, it seems feasible for all HCPs to assume everyone they treat has experienced trauma and apply trauma-informed care to all [30]. Even the fortunate patient who has never experienced an adverse physical, sexual, or other traumatic event will benefit from the provision of safe, non-judgmental care.

It is particularly important that trauma-informed care be provided in all health care settings where physical exams/procedures are routine such as obstetrics and gynecology, reproductive medicine, and urology clinics. Trauma-informed care in these clinics should include the routine private screening of patients for a history of sexual

Table 3.1 TIC Behaviors and Potential Benefits

TIC behaviors	Examples		Potential patient benefit
Develop trust first	• Take a history with patient during a clothed appointment separate and prior to any physical examination • Privately screen for the history of trauma at each appointment • Use language for body parts desired by the patient • Use appropriate patient pronouns and name • Provide non-judgmental counseling/support • Avoid stigmatizing/blame		• Increased: – Patient sense of control – Feelings of empowerment – Trust in HCP – Patient satisfaction – Treatment adherence – Patient uptake of mental health support – Promotion of healing and health – Probability of future disclosure of trauma – Shared decision making – Patient-centered care • Decreased: – Feelings of vulnerability – Avoidance of care – Re-traumatization – Physical pain during care – Triggering of psychological distress
Inform before perform	• Inform patients of all aspects of procedures before and throughout • Explain all steps of procedures • Show the instruments/room, etc. that will be used • Consent each step…and stop procedure if patient asks and it is safe		
Flexible care	• Offer appointments with female HCPs if desired and possible and if not, having a female HCP (e.g., nurse, ultrasonographer) in the room for all appointments • Allow a support person in the room • Do not have patient remove clothing if moving clothing aside is acceptable • Offer mirror to visualize during exam • Offer self-insertion of speculum • Ask patients what would increase comfort • Allow home semen collection		
Pain management	• Use lubrication where appropriate • Use smaller instruments • Offer abdominal versus internal exam • Do not invalidate pain by saying “it won’t hurt” or “it will be over soon” • Use warm instruments/room • Offer a blanket/socks		
Language	Avoid:	Consider:	
	– “Bed”	– “Table”	
	– “Stirrups”	– “Footrests”	
	– “Lube”	– “Lubricant”	
	– “Relax”	– “Some people find it helpful to take deep breaths during these exams”	
	– “Lay back”	– “So that I can start the exam, could you please lay with your back on the table?”	
	– “Spread your legs”	– “Can you please let your knees fall to the side like an open book?”	
	– “It won’t hurt”	– “Please let me know if you feel any pain or discomfort”	
	– “Don’t move”	– “I know this can be uncomfortable. Please let me know if you need to adjust your body”	
	– “It will be over soon”	– “Let me know if you need to take a break or if you are ok with me continuing the exam. Explain what else needs to be completed for the exam”	
	– Medical jargon		
	– Unnecessary questions		
Action	• Don’t: – Spread patient’s legs – Obscure your face – Set unrealistic expectations • Do: – Engage in annual TIC training – Recognize/respond to trauma reactions – Understand the health and other sequalae of trauma – Understand your reactions to trauma disclosure – Have ready access to trusted mental health professionals		

victimization by healthcare professionals who are sensitive to and non-judgmental of patient experiences, who understand the negative sequalae and common coping responses to such experiences (e.g., not formally reporting, substance use, engagement in other maladaptive coping), and who have the resources needed to support patients (e.g., referral to integrated mental health professional, other mental health supports) [1, 29]. Examples of trauma-informed care in such HCP settings include but are not limited to: (1) developing a trusting relationship with avoidance of victim-blaming and taking a history with the patient during a clothed appointment separate and prior to any physical examination, (2) informing patients of all aspects of procedures before and throughout the procedures, (3) being flexible in the provision of care, (4) attending to patient's experience of pain, (5) using appropriate language, and (6) engaging in supportive actions. Each of these trauma-informed behaviors are hypothesized to lead to the same mental and physical health benefits for patients (see Table 3.1 for examples of these behaviors and their potential benefits) [1, 29, 31].

Special Considerations in Reproductive Medicine

In reproductive medicine clinics vaginal/internal exams and procedures, the production of semen via masturbation, sexually transmitted infection testing, discussion related to intercourse and ejaculation, discussion of history of pregnancy loss and abortion, discovery of infertility due to a prior sexually transmitted infection or injury from sexual victimization, partners not being aware of each other's trauma histories and fear that they may be discovered during evaluation, patient loss of sense of control of their bodies and their ability to control their reproductive futures, and other potential trauma triggers are common. The focus on repeated touching of patient's bodies and discussions related to sex lives on a weekly if not daily basis (for months to years) for patients undergoing fertility evaluation and/or treatment is likely experienced more intensely than an annual exam with an ObGyn or other HCP. Infertility, pregnancy loss, surgery (e.g., hysterectomy, salpingectomy, testicular sperm extraction), and other negative reproductive-related events may be experienced as traumatic and be associated with trauma reactions and/or trigger past trauma experiences. In addition, it is not uncommon for patients to have a reproductive endocrinologist and infertility specialist (REI) who is not their primary REI conduct physical exams or procedures during receipt of fertility treatment. This REI may be male, other male HCPs (e.g., anesthesiologist, nurse) may be present during receipt of care, and the patient may have never met the HCP prior to the exam/procedure thereby preventing the patient from developing a trusting relationship with them. For LGBTQ+ patients and other patients who have been harmed by health care professionals (see, e.g., [8]) and/or they or their community targeted and stigmatized for who they are or who they love are likely to be fearful of how they will be treated in reproductive medicine clinics. Finally, individuals who have experienced sexual victimization have often been blamed for their experiences (e.g., what were you wearing, why were you drinking alcohol, why didn't you run away/fight back, why didn't you just quit, etc.) which adds to the psychological distress of the traumatic event(s) and leads to hesitancy in disclosing their experiences and associated emotional reactions [3, 32]. Historically, women in fertility settings have similarly been "victim-blamed" for their experiences of infertility or reproductive loss due to a supposed biologic role of stress in reproduction leading these women to suffer infertility and loss in silence. Given that there is no rigorous research that supports a biologic role of stress in reproduction and that blaming women for their difficulty conceiving is experienced as harmful to women struggling to cope with infertility and loss, it is vital that REIs and other HCPs in reproductive medicine clinics also avoid re-victimizing or triggering patients' previous experiences of being blamed for something beyond their control by inappropriately blaming them for their struggles [33]. In light of the multiple risks of re-traumatization of reproductive medicine patients, it is vital that all clinic members undergo repeated trauma-informed care training to prevent further harming patients and provide effective patient-centered care.

A word about "difficult" patients in REI. An important aspect of trauma-informed care in reproductive medicine includes the use of empathy when working with patients and their partners. At its core, empathy is about understanding that others might view the world and their experiences in an emotionally different way than you do and as a result responding to them in a supportive manner. Patients who are perceived as "difficult" are often described as emotionally reacting to the bad news (e.g., delays in care, need for third party reproduction, failed treatment cycles, pregnancy losses) they received from their clinic in a way that the healthcare professional finds distressing (e.g., the patient presents as angry, needy, anxious, or depressed). Given that most patients have experienced at least one kind of traumatic event in their lives and that many people have experienced sexual victimization that left them feeling helpless, it is not surprising that patients who face another potentially traumatizing event associated with a loss of sense of control in their lives (e.g., the inability to have a baby) would react with intense feelings of distress. Sadness, anger, anxiety and the need for validation and support in the setting of the unfairness of infertility and reproductive loss and the fear that they will not be able to be a parent is unavoidable. Patient-centered care and trauma-informed care require that HCPs attempt to uncover and understand why a patient is being "difficult" while setting boundaries for inappropriate behaviors. It is likely in the setting of reproductive medicine that the patient who is perceived to be "difficult" is actually a patient who has been or is feeling traumatized. Uncovering the cause of the patient's behavior can therefore help HCPs engage in greater empathy during the provision of trauma-informed care and thus promote patient healing and support.

Conclusions

Whether attempted or completed assault, sexual harassment or some other form of sexual violence, research shows that most women and many men have experienced sexual victimization in some form. These experiences of sexual victimization result in a heightened risk of numerous negative health, academic, occupational, relational, economic, and other outcomes and increases the likelihood that receipt of healthcare from male HCPs and/or healthcare which includes repeated touching of women's and men's bodies or a focus on sex and reproduction may be emotionally distressing. Receipt of healthcare may be increasingly distressing for survivors if the HCP further stigmatizes the patient for her/his experiences or responses to those experiences. It is therefore vital that all HCPs not only screen patients for a history of sexual victimization at every visit (as sexual victimization can occur at any time in a person's life) but also provide trauma-informed care to all patients (as sexual victimization is prevalent and as trauma-informed care is patient-centered care). Given the unique body and sex-focused nature of reproductive, gynecologic, and urologic healthcare, the provision of trauma-informed care in these patient populations is even more vital.

References

1. Raja S, Hasnain M, Hoersch M, Gove-Yin S, Rajagopalan C. Trauma informed care in medicine: current knowledge and future research directions. Fam Community Health. 2015;38(3):216–26.
2. Fitzgerald LF, Swan S, Magley VJ. But was it really sexual harassment? Legal, behavioral, and psychological definitions of the workplace victimization of women. In: O'Donohue W, editor. Sexual harassment, theory, research, and treatment. Boston, MA: Allyn and Bacon; 1997. p. 5–28.
3. Fitzgerald LF, Swan S, Fischer K. Why didn't she just report him? The psychological and legal implications of women's responses to sexual harassment. J Soc Issues. 1995;51:117–38.
4. Tjaden PG. Full report of the prevalence, incidence, and consequences of violence against women: findings from the national violence against women survey. In: Dept. of Justice, Office of Justice Programs, National Institute of Justice, editors. Washington, DC 2000.
5. Black MC, Basile KC, Breiding MJ, Smith SG, Walters ML, Merrick MT, et al. In: National Center for Injury Prevention and Control, editor. The National Intimate Partner and sexual violence survey (NISVS): 2010 summary report. Atlanta, GA: Centers for Disease Control and Prevention; 2011.
6. World Health Organization. Violence against women Prevalence Estimates, 2018. Global, regional and national prevalence estimates for intimate partner violence against women and global and regional prevalence estimates for non-partner sexual violence against women. Geneva, Switzerland: World Health Organization; 2021.
7. Walters ML, Chen J, Breiding MJ. In: National Center for Injury Prevention and Control, editor. The national intimate partner and sexual violence survey (NISVS): 2010 findings on victimization by sexual orientation. Atlanta, GA: Centers for Disease Control and Prevention; 2013.
8. James SE, Herman JL, Rankin S, Keisling M, Mottet L, Anafi M. The report of the 2015 U.S. transgender survey. Washington, DC: National Center for Transgender Equality; 2016.

9. Beck AJ, Berzofsky M, Caspar R, Krebs C. In: Department of Justice, editor. Sexual victimization in prisons and jails reported by inmates 2011–2012. Office of Justice Programs, Bureau of Justice Statistics; 2013.
10. Fedina L, Holmes JL, Backes BL. Campus sexual assault: a systematic review of prevalence research from 2000 to 2015. Trauma Violence Abuse. 2018;19(1):76–93.
11. Snyder JA, Fisher BS, Scherer HL, Daigle LE. Unsafe in the camouflage tower: sexual victimization and perceptions of military academy leadership. J Interpers Violence. 2012;27(16):3171–94.
12. Willness CR, Steel P, Lee K. A meta-analysis of the antecedents and consequences of workplace sexual harassment. Pers Psychol. 2007;60(1):127–62.
13. Smith SG, Chen J, Basile KC, Gilbert LK, Merrick MT, Patel N, et al. In: National Center for Injury Prevention and Control, editor. The national intimate partner and sexual violence survey (NISVS): 2010–2012 state report. Atlanta, GA: Centers for Disease Control and Prevention; 2017.
14. Smith SG, Zhang X, Basile KC, Merrick MT, Wang J, Kresnow M, et al. The national intimate partner and sexual violence survey (NISVS): 2015 data brief—updated release. In: National Center for Injury Prevention and Control, editor. . Atlanta, GA: Centers for Disease Control and Prevention; 2018.
15. Dworkin ER, Jaffe AE, Bedard-Gilligan M, Fitzpatrick S. PTSD in the year following sexual assault: a meta-analysis of prospective studies. Trauma Violence Abuse. 2023;24(2):497–514.
16. Molstad TD, Weinhardt JM, Jones R. Sexual assault as a contributor to academic outcomes in university: a systematic review. Trauma Violence Abuse. 2023;24(1):218–30.
17. Irish L, Kobayashi I, Delahanty DL. Long-term physical health consequences of childhood sexual abuse: a meta-analytic review. J Pediatr Psychol. 2010;35(5):450–61.
18. Ahrens CE, Alanda E. The ties that bind: understanding the impact of sexual assault disclosure on survivors' relationships with friends, family, and partners. J Trauma Dissociation. 2012;13:226–43.
19. Lorenz K, O'Callaghan E. 'I realized that I couldn't act Normal': a qualitative study of sexual assault survivors' experiences of workplace disclosure. J Fam Violence. 2022;37:381–93.
20. Dworkin ER, Menon SV, Bystrynski J, Allen NE. Sexual assault victimization and psychopathology: a review and meta-analysis. Clin Psychol Rev. 2017;56:65–81.
21. Loya RM. Rape as an economic crime: the impact of sexual violence on survivors' employment and economic well-being. J Interpers Violence. 2015;30(16):2793–813.
22. Fitzgerald LF, Drasgow F, Hulin CL, Gelfand MJ, Magley VJ. Antecedents and consequences of sexual harassment in organizations: a test of an integrated model. J Appl Psychol. 1997;82(4):578–89.
23. Lawson AK, Fitzgerald LF. Sexual harassment litigation: a road to re-victimization or recovery? Psychol Inj Law. 2016;9:216–29.
24. American Psychiatric Association. Diagnostic and statistical manual of mental disorders. 5th ed. Arlington, VA: American Psychiatric Association; 2013.
25. Farrow VA, Bosch J, Crawford JN, Snead C, Schulkin J. Screening for history of childhood abuse: beliefs, practice patterns, and barriers among obstetrician-gynecologists. Womens Health Issues. 2018;28(6):559–68.
26. Stevens NR, Tironea V, Lillis TA, Holmgreen L, Chen-McCracken A, Hobfoll SE. Posttraumatic stress and depression may undermine abuse survivors' self-efficacy in the obstetric care setting. J Psychosom Obstet Gynaecol. 2017;38:103–10.
27. Flanagan T, Alabaster A, McCaw B, Stoller N, Watson C, Young-Wolff KC. Feasibility and acceptability of screening for adverse childhood experiences in prenatal care. J Womens Health (Larchmt). 2018;27(7):903–11.
28. Berry KM, Rutledge CM. Factors that influence women to disclose sexual assault history to health care providers. J Obstet Gynecol Neonatal Nurs. 2016;45(4):553–64.
29. Havig K. The health care experiences of adult survivors of child sexual abuse: a systematic review of evidence on sensitive practice. Trauma Violence Abuse. 2008;9(1):19–33.

30. Felitti VJ, Anda RF, Nordenberg D, Williamson DF, Spitz AM, Edwards V, et al. Relationship of childhood abuse and household dysfunction to many of the leading causes of death in adults. The adverse childhood experiences (ACE) study. Am J Prev Med. 1998;14(4):245–58.
31. Ades V, Wu SX, Rabinowitz E, Chemouni Bach S, Goddard B, Pearson Ayala S, et al. An integrated, trauma-informed care model for female survivors of sexual violence: the engage, motivate, protect, organize, self-worth, educate, respect (EMPOWER). Clin Obstet Gynecol. 2019;133(4):803–9.
32. Thelan AR, Meadows, EA. The Illinois Rape Myth Acceptance Scale—Subtle Version: Using an Adapted Measure to Understand the Declining Rates of Rape Myth Acceptance. J Interpers Violence. 2022;37:19–20.
33. Lawson AK. Caution is warranted when discussing correlations between stress and reproductive outcomes. Fertil Steril. 2020;114(5):972–3.

Chapter 4
Trauma-Informed Care in Patients with a History of Medical Trauma

Amelia Swanson and Krithika Malhotra

Introduction

Medical diagnoses, procedures, and treatment can cause traumatic stress but are often overlooked by healthcare professionals and patients when considering traumatic events. For fertility patients, a history of medical trauma may be separate from their fertility issues, may be a reason for their infertility (e.g., Asherman's syndrome after a traumatic birth or D&C), and/or may be newly experienced during fertility treatment. A history of medical trauma and experiencing new medical traumas can lead patients to avoid medical treatment and/or treatment-related medications and to drop out at various points of treatment (e.g., when needing to give injections or have anesthesia) [1, 2]. Medical trauma can also lead to significant mistrust in medical systems and healthcare professionals which can impact a patient's behavior and interaction with the medical team [1].

Medical care which attends to the Substance Abuse and Mental Health Administration's (SAMHSA) [3] six key principles of trauma-informed care (safety; trustworthiness and transparency; peer support; collaboration and mutuality; empowerment, voice, and choice; cultural, historical, and gender issues) is imperative for all patients (given the high risk of childhood and adult traumas) but is particularly salient for patients with a history of medical trauma [4, 5]. Patients with a history of medical trauma have directly experienced one or more events

A. Swanson (✉)
Health Psychology Associates of Illinois PLLC, Skokie, IL, USA
e-mail: amelia@healthpsychologyillinois.com

K. Malhotra
Department of Family and Community Medicine, Feinberg School of Medicine, Northwestern University, Chicago, IL, USA
e-mail: krithika.malhotra@nm.org

A. Lawson, A. Swanson (eds.), *Trauma-Informed Reproductive Healthcare*, https://doi.org/10.1007/978-3-031-67474-7_4

wherein their safety was compromised, their trust in their healthcare professional or healthcare system was betrayed, they experienced discrimination based on their identity, and/or they felt disempowered and devalued during that experience. Developing trust in a new healthcare professional or organization in this context would be expected to be difficult, even impossible, if the healthcare professional/organization does not consistently and meaningfully engage in trauma-informed care.

Medical Trauma

Medical trauma "occurs from direct contact with the medical setting, and develops through a complex interaction between the patient, medical staff, medical environment, and the diagnostic and/or procedural experience that can have powerful psychological impacts due to the patient's unique interpretation of the event (p. 18) [6]." Medical trauma can result from a variety of medical experiences including the experience of a serious or chronic illness/diagnosis and adverse medical events [6]. It may also arise following the betrayal of trust when a patient experiences medical abuse (e.g., assault, fertility fraud) [7], discrimination and/or institutional betrayal (e.g., organizational actions or inactions which worsen the impact of traumatic experiences such as not taking seriously a patient's report of experiencing medical abuse or minimizing the emotional consequences of reproductive clinic errors) [8, 9] as harm perpetrated by individuals and organizations that are believed to be trustworthy may be considered traumatic by patients. Medical trauma is thus directly tied to the medical environment and medical staff and may occur at any point in an individual's life. For example, research finds that most adults with symptoms of needle phobia and dental phobia developed these anxious symptoms in childhood following a traumatic experience receiving an injection at the dentist [10].

A key aspect to medical trauma is the relational aspect of the patient-healthcare professional relationship [6]. The patient-healthcare professional relationship is hierarchical with the healthcare professional having more power than the patient. Therefore, the patient must have some level of trust in the healthcare professional to accept their care. Any experience of medical trauma threatens that sense of trust and safety in any healthcare professional (HCP) as well as the medical system. Some experiences of medical trauma are the direct result of the HCP's behaviors and choices, such as not respecting consent, making medical errors, and assault/discrimination [11]. Other experiences of medical trauma may occur even if the HCP upheld all ethical and practice standards but still was unable to prevent a medical emergency, pain or suffering.

Medical trauma is also frequently disenfranchised, or not socially acknowledged or recognized [12]. For example, people that have experienced birth trauma with severe complications and near-death experiences are often told by family, friends, and even their HCP that their traumatic experience was not that bad because they survived and have a healthy baby. Disenfranchised trauma is especially difficult because it can lead to feelings of isolation and invalidation, compound the experience of trauma, and prolong the experience of distress [12].

It is difficult to quantify the rates and prevalence of medical trauma due to the varied nature of diagnoses and procedures that patients' experience. Despite this, there are a few specific medical procedures/events as well as medical conditions that have been found to have the highest risk for the development of PTSD. In terms of medical conditions, burns have been found to be most associated with PTSD diagnoses, secondary to the painful experience of the injury, extended hospital stays and outpatient care, painful procedures and daily care needed, high contact with medical professionals, and possibility for complications during recovery may all be traumatizing [13].

Intraoperative awareness and Intensive Care Unit (ICU) stay are medical procedures/experiences that have been found to be associated with the highest rates of PTSD compared to other medical experiences [13]. Patients experiencing both intraoperative awareness and ICU stay likely have an inability to move and loss of power during the experience which may be particularly distressing. ICU admission also likely includes the experience of prolonged hospitalization which may include complications due to the illness/event or due to medical errors/miscommunications [13]. Even though fertility patients are unlikely to be hospitalized during treatment, being in a medical setting, interacting with medical professionals, being in procedure spaces or being in a fertility clinic on a medical campus may all be triggering for someone with a history of prolonged hospitalization due to birth trauma, serious injury, or other medical issue. It is important to note that PTSD rates for patients with medical trauma have been found to remain stable over time for some after the medical event, indicating that the amount of time after the medical event is not necessarily associated with the level of distress [13].

For patients who have experienced medical trauma prior to contact with a fertility clinic, fertility treatment is likely to have some similarities to previous traumatic medical experiences such as a loss of sense of control and power, pain, intrusive medical procedures, feelings of fear, and a focus on sexual behaviors. There can be concrete similarities such as the appointment occurring in the same medical complex as a prior trauma; having similar furniture/decorations, smells or sounds as the office wherein a prior trauma occurred; or having an HCP of the same sex or race as the individual who engaged in prior medical abuse. The similarities could be more abstract such as a familiar power differential where the patient has less power than an HCP or the patient generally feeling out of control or scared. Due to these likely similarities, fertility treatment can be a reminder or trigger for a previous traumatic medical experience.

Fertility patients who have experienced prior medical trauma may also be more attuned to any risks of fertility treatment as hypervigilance related to their safety during medical care is heightened. Given that medical traumas may be perceived as low probability events, patients may be more concerned about fertility treatment complications than an average patient as even a complication with a low rate of occurrence may seem very possible, if not likely, to happen to them.

Type of Medical Traumas Relevant to Fertility Patients

Before beginning to talk about different types of medical trauma, it is important to note that marginalized patients, such as LGBTQ+ patients and patients of color, are more likely to experience a number of health issues, be less believed about pain, experience medical and social discrimination or harassment, and to experience increased rates of morbidity and threat of mortality around giving birth [4, 11, 14]. Therefore, it is important to keep in mind that LGBTQ+ patients and patients of color may be particularly and reasonably attuned to the lack of trauma-informed care, possible medical discrimination and microaggressions, and may be vigilant for the realistic possibility of traumatic or dangerous experiences.

Painful and/or Invasive Gynecological Exams/Procedures Many common gynecological exams are similar to exams in fertility treatment (e.g., transvaginal exams, use of speculums, and laying on exam tables with footrests). The similarities between gynecological and fertility procedures may trigger memories of painful exams or make the patient expect that the fertility exam/procedure will be traumatic. Fertility exams and procedures can also be intensely distressing for patients who have experienced sexual or physical abuse at the hands of a HCP or other individual. Finally, given many women's history of not being believed about their experience of pain during receipt of Ob/Gyn care, they may feel disempowered to share their experience of pain during vaginal exams, following oocyte retrieval (see, e.g., "The Retrievals") or during intrauterine insemination or embryo transfer procedures [15, 16].

Unexpected Surgical Outcomes Fertility patients may have had prior surgeries with unexpected diagnoses or outcomes. For example, this could be from a poor outcome of an orthopedic surgery that may need multiple revisions in order to heal, an emergency hysterectomy following delivery of a prior child, or from a biopsy with a diagnosis of cancer that was unexpected. This is also common in fertility patients that may have had negative outcomes from surgeries such as surgery for endometriosis or fibroids, cancer surgery or biopsy, unexpected outcomes from D&C (e.g., Asherman's syndrome), emergency salpingectomy following an ectopic pregnancy, or complications associated with oocyte stimulation and/or retrieval (e.g., ovarian torsion, OHSS, perforated bladder, infection).

Unexpected Medical Issues/Diagnoses Many fertility patients may have gone in for a prior routine medical appointment only to receive a diagnosis that was a surprise or a shock such as someone going into a medical appointment for a sore back who gets diagnosed with a lifelong autoimmune disorder. Similarly, patients may be shocked to learn at a routine annual Ob/Gyn visit that they likely have cancer, are infertile, or are carriers for a genetic disorder. Other patients may have been told at prior medical visits that a certain problem was unlikely to happen, such as an ectopic pregnancy or ovarian torsion following IVF, only to experience this low probability event themselves. This may lead patients to not be comforted by statistics of low rates of occurrence of a negative event, hypervigilance related to their medical safety, and distrust of medical professionals.

Difficult Interactions with Medical Team Patients may have experienced a variety of difficult interactions while undergoing medical treatment, including being dismissed, criticized, their concerns minimized or even not feeling confident in the medical team's competency. Long wait times and short appointment slots are common in the US healthcare system which can also lead to a lack of trust and feeling abandoned at a vulnerable time. This can lead patients to prepare for contentious medical appointments and perceive ambiguous situations as purposely harmful due to medical cynicism [17].

Weight bias, or discrimination based on overweight/obesity, is a common type of difficult interaction for patients. Patients report weight bias occurring in medical settings frequently from all types of medical professionals [18]. Research shows that physicians are more likely to focus on weight loss for patients who are obese even when they come in to address a very different issue [19]. Obesity is a known risk factor for infertility and pregnancy loss and fertility clinics often have BMI cut offs for IVF or other fertility procedures [20, 21]. As a result, patients may be likely to expect weight bias during fertility treatment and may be sensitive to a medical professional's focus on weight [22]. Patients may feel blamed by their HCP for their infertility or pregnancy loss because of the belief that obese patients are entirely responsible for their weight, despite extensive research indicating that even intensive behavioral lifestyle changes lead to minimal weight loss [23]. Patients who have experienced verbal abuse or who have been denied care due to their weight may also fear similar experiences during receipt of fertility care.

Anesthesia Ineffectiveness Intraoperative awareness is likely to include feelings of pain, loss of control, anxiety, and panic [13]. In addition, due to the medications used in anesthesia, patients may feel pain but be unable to move or communicate to their medical team. In certain procedures or due to the anesthesia, patients may also be intubated which can be uncomfortable and frightening. Intraoperative awareness can occur in many settings including medical or dental settings, in operating rooms in hospitals or outpatient procedure rooms. This is particularly relevant to fertility patients as they are likely to have procedures requiring anesthesia during egg retrievals, hysteroscopy procedures, and D&Cs.

Fertility patients may be particularly attuned to intraoperative awareness or poor pain control post egg retrieval following the well-publicized events at Yale fertility clinic in 2023. It has been reported that a nurse in that fertility clinic was diverting pain medication, leaving patients in pain during and after procedures for many months before being discovered [24]. In addition to the experience of medical abuse, it has also been reported that many affected patients experienced institutional betrayal when they experienced invalidating responses by their healthcare team at Yale following their complaints of experiencing pain during their retrievals. This was national news at the time that the nurse was arrested and was further publicized by a podcast by Serial Productions and The New York Times called Retrievals that chronicled this event.

Chronic Pain/Illness Fertility patients may be coping with a number of chronic illnesses which can be traumatic. History of chronic or acute disease is a risk factor for PTSD [25]. Chronic illnesses and/or chronic pain may be difficult to manage and often require frequent interactions with the medical system which may expose patients to additional traumatic experiences [13]. Chronic pain is an often difficult to treat medical issue and patients may have a history of difficult medical interactions including being disbelieved, dismissed or accused of having an addiction. Additionally, pain can be exacerbated by stressful events, such as ongoing fertility issues and fertility treatment. Furthermore, people who are on long-term pain medications, including long-term NSAID use, may need to discontinue their medication for fertility treatment and pregnancy and patients with long-term opiate use may be difficult to sedate for an egg retrieval or to manage additional pain after a procedure. All of these issues may make a patient with chronic pain and/or medical management of pain more likely to be hypervigilant during the fertility process as they may fear the consequences of medication changes, impact of fertility treatment on their pain, or new medical trauma during fertility treatment (e.g., sedation ineffectiveness).

Pregnancy/Childbirth Fertility patients may have a history of a traumatic birth or pregnancy which could contribute to their need for fertility treatment. Other patients may have secondary infertility due to medical complications during birth such as Asherman's syndrome or may need to collaborate with a gestational carrier or other third-party reproduction collaborator due to complications during pregnancy or birth. Pregnancy and birth trauma are not uncommon; one meta-analysis found that approximately 3.3% of births resulted in PTSD, and up to 18.95% of high-risk births resulted in PTSD [26]. Birth trauma can be associated with events that are significantly life-threatening to the patient or their baby that oftentimes may have been unexpected. It can also arise following experiences that from a medical perspective were low to moderate risk but from a patient's perspective seemed highly dangerous. Although there are limited data about the experience of traumatic pregnancies, the experience of hyperemesis gravitas or other serious pregnancy complications can be experienced as traumatic for patients [26]. Finally, some patients may believe they have recovered from a traumatic pregnancy/birth experience only to be emotionally triggered by receiving care in a fertility clinic as it can be a reminder of past experiences and the possibility of a subsequent pregnancy/birth and all the risks that entails.

Fertility patients who have experienced prior sexual or physical assault by Ob/Gyns [27] or other HCPs (e.g., Larry Nasser) may be more likely to be worried about being re-traumatized with news of alleged medical fraud by fertility physicians using their own sperm for treatments. Deemed "fertility fraud," the first instance of medical deception related to fertility treatment was described to have occurred in 1884 when a female patient was sedated under the guise of conducting a minor procedure and donor sperm was inserted into her uterus without her consent [28]. With the popularity of personal DNA testing, numerous additional instances of fertility fraud have and likely will continue to be discovered [29]. These instances of fertility fraud and highly publicized cases of alleged fertility clinic errors are likely to increase patient fears of such experiences.

Medical Trauma During Fertility Treatment

Many patients arrive at fertility clinics with medical trauma, but others unfortunately experience medical trauma for the first-time while receiving fertility treatment. Although trauma is based on personal experience and is subjective, there are some events that are known to be more likely to be traumatic for fertility patients. Medical events that are commonly experienced as traumatic for fertility patients including painful transvaginal exams/ultrasounds, SIS, HSG, unexpected diagnoses or outcomes, pregnancy loss, lab or other clinic errors, treatment failures, and medical/surgical complications.

Transvaginal Exams and Ultrasounds These procedures may be traumatic for fertility patients due to their intimate nature, lack of control by the patient, and possibility for pain or discomfort. Patients that have not previously had intercourse or utilized tampons, feel anxious about the exam, have experienced sexual assault, or have not had previous pelvic exams may be especially at risk for experiencing transvaginal exams as traumatic. Saline ultrasounds can be traumatic for similar reasons as transvaginal exams and ultrasounds: due to their intimate nature, lack of control by patients, and pain or discomfort. Different from transvaginal ultrasounds, they are more likely to be painful for patients, which may be a surprise to them.

HSGs are often experienced as painful by patients, although this experience varies widely [30]. Many patients report that the dye that is inserted into their uterus causes extreme pain and intense cramping. Although the feeling does not last long, it can be extreme; and their experience may be worsened by a HCP who uses language which invalidates their pain or mirrors language that may have been used by a past rapist (e.g., “this won’t hurt,” “it will be over soon,” “don’t move”). Finally, patients may not be told about possible pain with HSGs as it can vary widely between patients and may not be offered evidence-based pain management options [30].

Pregnancy Loss Fertility patients often experience pregnancy loss which is traumatic for many patients. After a history of infertility or pregnancy loss, patients are often hopeful that subsequent pregnancies (especially those beginning after fertility treatment) will be viable, and therefore can be devastated to learn of a subsequent pregnancy loss. Patients are also often seen for early ultrasounds at fertility clinics and thus may be more likely to find out about the pregnancy loss at the fertility clinic. In turn, later visits to the clinic, ultrasound room or other aspects of the fertility treatment strongly associated with a traumatic event are likely to trigger emotional distress. Other patients may not expect a pregnancy loss because their embryos were genetically tested and found to be chromosomally normal prior to a transfer and these patients may feel especially helpless and shocked by the loss.

Fertility patients are often relatively healthy people who do not expect to have fertility challenges. They are often physically active with a healthy diet and limited smoking and alcohol consumption. Some fertility patients have had children previously so understandably do not expect to have fertility problems. Fertility patients are often surprised by unexpected diagnoses for even common types of infertility. Patients with little history of pain or who have been reassured that their pain was normal, may be shocked to find out they have stage IV endometriosis. Other patients may have less common medical or genetic conditions that are shocking to them and shake their trust in their own bodies, health and possibility of having genetically related children in the future.

Other patients may have unexpected outcomes to fertility treatment. Patients may not respond well to fertility medications (e.g., have a large number of eggs at retrieval) despite normal testing and a young age, others may be surprised to have empty follicles, lack of fertilization of eggs, poor-quality embryos, or unsuccessful repeated transfer of euploid embryos. These outcomes can be especially difficult as patients may have been reassured by their medical team that they were likely to have a good response to treatment.

Medical or Surgical Complications Although fertility treatments have been widely studied and found to be relatively safe to engage in, they are not without risk. For example, contradictory research exists with regard to the risk of repeated hormone exposure and the development of cancer; some research findings show that a diagnosis of infertility rather than infertility treatment is associated with this heightened risk [31, 32]. Similarly contradictory research exists related to the risks to children being conceived through fertility treatment [33]; overall this research shows that risks to fertility treatment conceived children are small. However, patients who develop cancer during or after engagement in fertility treatment may fear that their treatment caused their condition. Surgical complications from fertility care or procedures are generally low and include but are not limited to risk of infection, emergency procedures such as oophorectomy or salpingectomy (e.g., following ovarian torsion or ectopic pregnancy), ovarian hyperstimulation syndrome (OHSS), perforations during surgery, bleeding, and pain [34]. Patients who experience a complication resulting from engagement in fertility treatment or related surgery may be shocked to learn they have experienced a low probability but potentially life or fertility threatening procedure.

Lab/Medical Errors Medical errors in a lab can vary widely and include minor errors in reporting lab values, errors in scheduling appointments, to much more significant medical errors such as destroying embryos in error, or fertilizing the wrong egg with the wrong sperm [35]. Sometimes even minor medical errors may make a patient question if this small mistake was why the cycle was not successful, such as a patient given wrong timing instructions for starting progesterone for her transfer cycle, or the wrong dose of stimulation medication for a night or two. Medical errors can be especially difficult for fertility patients if they have a history of medical trauma, poor treatment or discrimination, or are from a group that historically has experienced medical discrimination. Fertility patients feel a lack of control and need to trust their medical teams with complex treatment decisions and courses, so experiencing an error can quickly erode that trust or trigger similar feelings to previous medical trauma.

There have been an increasing number of lawsuits related to fertility lab errors/adverse events such as alleged tank failures that have resulted in loss of or potential damage to frozen eggs, embryos, and sperm, but there are undoubtedly numerous other similar errors that have been settled prior to public lawsuits. Patient awareness of these cases may heighten their concerns about their care in the fertility clinic.

Impacts of Medical Trauma on Fertility Treatment

Previous and ongoing medical trauma can have a wide range of effects on fertility patients, staff, healthcare professionals, and clinics. After financial reasons, stress is a main cause of patients dropping out of fertility treatment prior to reaching their family building goals [36]. Medical trauma may contribute to the overall experience of stress that fertility patients experience and may lead them to avoid, postpone, or drop out of treatment. Specifically, patients may not seek out treatment or avoid treatment due to similarities in medical settings (small consult rooms with no windows, short appointment times, rushed staff, pictures of babies on the walls, limited forms or artwork which resemble the patient's identities, etc.). Being in a similar setting could be triggering of symptoms of PTSD, anxiety, depression, and general stress and therefore patients may avoid treatment.

In addition to avoiding treatment, patients may also be perceived as difficult, demanding or controlling due to their history of medical trauma. They may be seeking care which mimics SAMHSA's 6 aspects of trauma-informed care by (1) trying to increase their sense of ***safety*** when interacting with the medical system, (2) assessing clinic ***transparency and accountability*** by attending to the clinics' acceptance of responsibility for mistaken scheduling and the like, (3) seeking ***collaboration*** and shared decision-making through questioning medical decisions, (4) ***empowering*** themselves to ask to re-check results or recommendations or seek out second, third or more opinions particularly due to lack of trust when (5) ***cultural or other concerns*** are not respected or they experience discrimination, and (6) assessing the level of ***peer support*** available through the clinic.

Practical Tips

Fertility clinics have the opportunity to support patients with a history of medical trauma and prevent new occurrences of medical trauma. Given the widespread prevalence of trauma, it is essential to incorporate trauma-informed care as a universal precaution to best serve the needs of all patients. Key assumptions (SAMHSA's fours R's) to consider when developing a trauma-informed approach include **realization** that trauma has a widespread impact on patients and their families, **recognition** of signs and symptoms of trauma in patients, clinic staff and HCPs, **responding** to the widespread impact of trauma by developing policies, procedures, and practices that integrate knowledge about trauma, and **resisting re-traumatization** in patients, staff, and HCPs [3]. Additionally, consideration of SAMHSA's six principles of trauma-informed care can aid in the development of a framework along with strategies to support patients and prevent new traumas [37].

Safety

- Design layout of clinic space and exam/ultrasound rooms to give patients a sense of safety. Be mindful of patients having easy access to door if needed. Ensure patients have sufficient privacy. Design the clinic space to be as warm, relaxing and comfortable as possible with artwork and clinic forms which include diverse identities.
- Allow and encourage support people to be engaged in visits in person or by phone.
- Offer options to be interviewed alone (e.g., support staff care for accompanying children).
- Have a chaperone in the room for all pelvic procedures per ACOG guidelines.

Trustworthiness and Transparency

- Acknowledge any errors with a clear corrective plan and strategies to prevent similar errors in the future.
- Direct discussion with written information of chances of success for all procedures including IUI, IVF, and use of donor gametes.
- Discussion of risks of procedures/treatments in clear and straightforward terms. Give patients written information regarding risks as well so they have time to process information and ask questions later.
- Describe ways in which an examination/procedure might interact with senses (e.g., you may hear a click when the speculum is opened, you may feel pressure or a warm sensation).

Peer Support

- Provide embedded support groups and access to embedded mental health professionals. If this is not possible, cultivate strong relationships with local support group leaders and mental health professionals that specialize in fertility issues.
- Clinics can collaborate with Resolve (www.resolve.org) or other patient advocacy groups to host events, support groups or facilitate referrals for patients.

Collaboration and Mutuality

- Include a thorough discussion of treatment options and recommendations while collaborating with the patient to incorporate their desires, goals, preferences as central aspects to their decision-making process.
- Ask patients for permission before any step of the physical exam and/or procedure.
- Use suggestive instead of instructive language (e.g. instead of "Take a deep breath for this part," say "Some people find it helpful to take a deep breath during this part of the exam."

Empowerment, Voice, and Choice

- Check in with patients about any concerns, fears, or questions about the exam/procedure before performing it.
- Ensure that HCPs and staff are actively respecting patient's consent, including allowing the patient to dictate the pace and listening to patient's verbal or non-verbal communication if they want to take a break from or discontinue the exam/procedure.

Respect and Acknowledgment in Cultural, Historical, and Gender Issues

- Provide ongoing training for cultural humility and competence for staff and HCPs.
- Value diversity in cultural backgrounds and beliefs during hiring and promotion practices.
- Be aware of clinic artwork and marketing to be inclusive of a diverse patient population.
- If using a language interpreter, consider the patient's gender and/or cultural preference for an interpreter.

Summary

Medical trauma is often not recognized by medical professionals as well as patients but is especially important for medical clinics to consider. REI patients may have a history of medical trauma that is tied to their experience of ongoing fertility issues, such as a traumatic birth or previous miscarriage. Furthermore, REI patients may experience a new medical trauma during the course of their fertility treatment, particularly if TIC practices are not implemented and maintained. REI patients are likely to be reminded of a previous medical trauma during fertility treatment. REI professionals can support patients through use of TIC practices to support patients by minimizing reminders of previous medical trauma, increase patient's sense of safety in the REI clinics, and reduce likelihood of new medical traumas.

References

1. Favaro A, Gerosa G, Caforio AL, Volpe B, Rupolo G, Zarneri D, Boscolo S, Pavan C, Tenconi E, d'Agostino C, Moz M, Torregrossa G, Feltrin G, Gambino A, Santonastaso P. Posttraumatic stress disorder and depression in heart transplantation recipients: the relationship with outcome and adherence to medical treatment. Gen Hosp Psychiatry. 2011;33(1):1–7. https://doi.org/10.1016/j.genhosppsych.2010.10.001.
2. Vika M, Raadal M, Skaret E, Kvale G. Dental and medical injections: prevalence of self-reported problems among 18-yr-old subjects in Norway. Eur J Oral Sci. 2006;114(2):122–7. https://doi.org/10.1111/j.1600-0722.2006.00335.x.
3. SAMHSA. SAMHSA's concept of truama and guidance for a trauma-informed approach. In (Vol. HHS Publication No. (SMA) 14–4884). Rockville, MD: Substance Abuse and Mental Health Services Administration 2014.
4. Merrick MT, Ford DC, Ports KA, Guinn AS. Prevalence of adverse childhood experiences from the 2011-2014 behavioral risk factor surveillance system in 23 states. JAMA Pediatr. 2018;172(11):1038–44. https://doi.org/10.1001/jamapediatrics.2018.2537.
5. Ogle CM, Rubin DC, Berntsen D, Siegler IC. The frequency and impact of exposure to potentially traumatic events over the life course. Clin Psychol Sci. 2013;1(4):426–34. https://doi.org/10.1177/2167702613485076.
6. Hall MF, Hall SE. Managing the psychological impact of medical trauma: a guide for mental health and health care professionals. New York, NY: Springer Publishing Co; 2017.
7. DuBois JM, Walsh HA, Chibnall JT, Anderson EE, Eggers MR, Fowose M, Ziobrowski H. Sexual violation of patients by physicians: a mixed-methods, exploratory analysis of 101 cases. Sex Abus. 2019;31(5):503–23. https://doi.org/10.1177/1079063217712217.
8. Shires DA, Jaffee K. Factors associated with health care discrimination experiences among a national sample of female-to-male transgender individuals. Health Soc Work. 2015;40(2):134–41. https://doi.org/10.1093/hsw/hlv025.
9. Smith CP, Freyd JJ. Institutional betrayal. Am Psychol. 2014;69(6):575–87. https://doi.org/10.1037/a0037564.
10. Orenius T, LicPsych, Säilä H, Mikola K, Ristolainen L. Fear of injections and needle phobia among children and adolescents: an overview of psychological, behavioral, and contextual factors. SAGE Open Nurs. 2018;4:2377960818759442. https://doi.org/10.1177/2377960818759442.
11. Vedam S, Stoll K, Taiwo TK, Rubashkin N, Cheyney M, Strauss N, McLemore M, Cadena M, Nethery E, Rushton E, Schummers L, Declercq E. The giving voice to mothers study: ineq-

uity and mistreatment during pregnancy and childbirth in the United States. Reprod Health. 2019;16(1):77. https://doi.org/10.1186/s12978-019-0729-2.
12. Doka KJ. Disenfranchised grief: new directions, challenges, and strategies for practice. Champaign, Ill: Research Press; 2002.
13. Cyr S, Guo X, Marcil MJ, Dupont P, Jobidon L, Benrimoh D, Guertin MC, Brouillette J. Posttraumatic stress disorder prevalence in medical populations: a systematic review and meta-analysis. Gen Hosp Psychiatry. 2021;69:81–93. https://doi.org/10.1016/j.genhosppsych.2021.01.010.
14. Baciu A, Negussie Y, Geller A, Weinstein JN, editors. Communities in action: pathways to health equity. The National Academies Press; 2017.
15. Boring BL, Walsh KT, Ng BW, Schlegel RJ, Mathur VA. Experiencing pain invalidation is associated with under-reporting of pain: a social psychological perspective on acute pain communication. J Pain. 2023; https://doi.org/10.1016/j.jpain.2023.11.011.
16. Grundström H, Engman L, Rimhagen E, Söderstierna C, Flink I. Experiences of communication in women with endometriosis: perceived validation and invalidation in different contexts, and associations with health-related quality of life. J Psychosom Obstet Gynaecol. 2023;44(1):2264483. https://doi.org/10.1080/0167482X.2023.2264483.
17. Jaiswal J, Halkitis PN. Towards a more inclusive and dynamic understanding of medical mistrust informed by science. Behav Med. 2019;45(2):79–85. https://doi.org/10.1080/08964289.2019.1619511.
18. Puhl RM, Brownell KD. Confronting and coping with weight stigma: an investigation of overweight and obese adults. Obesity. 2006;14(10):1802–15. https://doi.org/10.1038/oby.2006.208.
19. Puhl RM, Phelan SM, Nadglowski J, Kyle TK. Overcoming weight bias in the management of patients with diabetes and obesity. Clin Diabetes. 2016;34(1):44–50. https://doi.org/10.2337/diaclin.34.1.44.
20. Hughes LM, McQueen DB, Jungheim ES, Merrion K, Boots CE. Maternal body mass index is not associated with increased rates of maternal embryonic aneuploidy. Fertil Steril. 2022;117(4):783. https://doi.org/10.1016/j.fertnstert.2021.12.031.
21. Turner-McGrievy GM, Grant BL. Prevalence of body mass index and body weight cut-off points for in vitro fertilization treatment at U.S. clinics and current clinic weight loss strategy recommendations. Hum Fertil. 2015;18(3):215–9. https://doi.org/10.3109/14647273.2015.1022606.
22. Evans AT, Vitek WS. Weight bias in reproductive medicine: a curiously unexplored frontier. Semin Reprod Med. 2023;41(3–04):63. https://doi.org/10.1055/s-0043-1777016.
23. Twells LK, Harris Walsh K, Blackmore A, Adey T, Donnan J, Peddle J, Ryan D, Farrell A, Nguyen H, Gao Z, Pace D. Nonsurgical weight loss interventions: a systematic review of systematic reviews and meta-analyses. Obes Rev. 2021;22(11):e13320. https://doi.org/10.1111/obr.13320.
24. Lindner E. The reverberations of pain and its dismissal. The New York Times, Section A, 2023 2. https://www.nytimes.com/2023/06/29/insider/the-reverberations-of-pain-and-its-dismissal.html.
25. Tortella-Feliu M, Fullana MA, Pérez-Vigil A, Torres X, Chamorro J, Littarelli SA, Solanes A, Ramella-Cravaro V, Vilar A, González-Parra JA, Andero R, Reichenberg A, Mataix-Cols D, Vieta E, Fusar-Poli P, Ioannidis JPA, Stein MB, Radua J, Fernández de la Cruz L. Risk factors for posttraumatic stress disorder: an umbrella review of systematic reviews and meta-analyses. Neurosci Biobehav Rev. 2019;107:154–65. https://doi.org/10.1016/j.neubiorev.2019.09.013.
26. Yildiz PD, Ayers S, Phillips L. The prevalence of posttraumatic stress disorder in pregnancy and after birth: a systematic review and meta-analysis. J Affect Disord. 2017;208:634–45. https://doi.org/10.1016/j.jad.2016.10.009.
27. Newhall K. The girls: an all-American Town, a predatory doctor, and the untold story of the gymnasts who brought him down by Pesta Abigail, and: start by believing: Larry Nasser's crimes, the institutions that enabled him, and the brave women who stopped a monster by Barr

John and Murphy Dan (review). Mich Hist Rev. 2021;47(1):132–6. https://doi.org/10.1353/mhr.2021.0017.
28. Braverman AM. How the internet is reshaping assisted reproduction: from donor offspring registries to direct-to-consumer genetic testing. Minn JL Sci Tech. 2010;11:477.
29. Madeira JL. Understanding illicit insemination and fertility fraud, from patient experience to legal reform. Columbia J Gend Law. 2020;39(1):110–204.
30. Unlu BS, Yilmazer M, Koken G, Arioz DT, Unlu E, Dogan Baki E, Kurttay C, Karacin O. Comparison of four different pain relief methods during hysterosalpingography: a randomized controlled study. Pain Res Manage. 2015;20(2):107–11. https://doi.org/10.1155/2015/306248.
31. Vassard D, Pinborg A, Kamper-Jørgensen M, Lyng Forman J, Glazer CH, Kroman N, Schmidt L. Assisted reproductive technology treatment and risk of breast cancer: a population-based cohort study. Hum Reprod. 2021;36(12):3152–60. https://doi.org/10.1093/humrep/deab219.
32. Vassard D, Schmidt L, Glazer CH, Lyng Forman J, Kamper-Jørgensen M, Pinborg A. Assisted reproductive technology treatment and risk of ovarian cancer—a nationwide population-based cohort study. Hum Reprod. 2019;34(11):2290–6. https://doi.org/10.1093/humrep/dez165.
33. Venetis C, Choi SKY, Jorm L, Zhang X, Ledger W, Lui K, Harvard A, Chapman M, Norman R, Chambers GM. Risk for congenital anomalies in children conceived with medically assisted fertility treatment: a population-based cohort study. Ann Intern Med. 2023;176(10):1308–20. https://doi.org/10.7326/M23-0872.
34. Klemetti R, Sevón T, Gissler M, Hemminki E. Complications of IVF and ovulation induction. Hum Reprod. 2005;20(12):3293–300. https://doi.org/10.1093/humrep/dei253.
35. Ifenatuoha CW, Mohammed C, Malhotra K. Errors in IVF laboratories: risks assessments and mitigations. Middle East Fertil Soc J. 2023;28(1):5. https://doi.org/10.1186/s43043-023-00130-0.
36. Gameiro S, Boivin J, Peronace L, Verhaak CM. Why do patients discontinue fertility treatment? A systematic review of reasons and predictors of discontinuation in fertility treatment. Hum Reprod Update. 2012;18(6):652–69. https://doi.org/10.1093/humupd/dms031.
37. Ravi A, Little V. Providing trauma-informed care. Am Fam Physician. 2017;95(10):655–7.

Chapter 5
Trauma-Informed Care in the Reproductive Clinical Setting for LGBTQ+ Patients

Colin B. Russell, Nicholas S. Raja, and Molly B. Moravek

Introduction: A Primer on Language

The LGBTQ+ (lesbian, gay, bisexual, transgender, queer) community is an expansive and diverse group encompassing people that identify outside the "traditional" boundaries of heterosexuality and the gender binary. Previously denoted simply as LGBT, the terms "queer," "plus," or simply "+," have been added for recognition of the unique nuances and variations that exist along the spectrums of gender and sexuality. A 2022 national survey of over 10,000 adults in the USA found that 7.2% of respondents identified as LGBTQ+, over twice that reported by a similar poll in 2012 [1]. Furthermore, the proportion of adults identifying as LGBTQ+ appears to be higher in younger generations, likely the result of increased visibility and acceptability over the last several decades. From this national poll, nearly 20% of adults from Generation Z (born between 1997 and 2014) identify as LGBTQ+ or non-heterosexual, compared with 2.7% of the Baby Boomer generation (born between 1946 and 1964) [1]. According to the Centers for Disease Control and Prevention, about 40% of the transgender population is younger than 25 years [2]. Given these findings, it will continue to be increasingly important that all healthcare professionals are able to deliver high-quality care to sexual and gender minority populations.

Best practice care begins with appropriate language. The terms "sex," "gender," "gender identity," "gender expression," and "sexual orientation" communicate distinct facets about a person's identity and are often misused [3, 4].

C. B. Russell (✉) · N. S. Raja
Department of Obstetrics and Gynecology, University of Michigan, Ann Arbor, MI, USA
e-mail: coru@med.umich.edu; nickraja@med.umich.edu

M. B. Moravek
Department of Obstetrics and Gynecology, University of Michigan, Ann Arbor, MI, USA

Department of Urology, University of Michigan, Ann Arbor, MI, USA

A. Lawson, A. Swanson (eds.), *Trauma-Informed Reproductive Healthcare*,
https://doi.org/10.1007/978-3-031-67474-7_5

A person's **sex** or **sex assigned at birth** refers to the classification of a person based on chromosomal makeup or external genitalia. Examples of sex include male, female, or intersex. In the literature, these terms are referred to as **Assigned Male At Birth (AMAB)** or **Assigned Female At Birth (AFAB)**.

The World Health Organization defines **gender** as characteristics of people that are socially constructed based on their sex assigned at birth, including "norms, behaviors, and roles" associated with the male and female sex [3]. Gender is distinct from, but interacts with, sex. **Gender identity** refers to the deeply felt, internal sense of being a female/woman, male/man, both of these, neither of these, or anything in between. For transgender and gender diverse individuals, their sex assigned at birth is incongruent with their gender identity. Examples of gender or gender identity include woman, man, girl, and boy, agender, gender-fluid, or gender non-binary.

Gender expression describes an individual's outward manifestation of their gender identity. Components of gender expression can include physical attributes (e.g., body shape or vocal tone) or stylistic choices (e.g., clothing or hairstyle).

Sexual orientation describes the relationship between a person's own gender identity and the gender identity/-ies of those to whom they are physically or emotionally attracted. Examples of sexual orientation include heterosexual/gay/lesbian, bisexual, asexual, pansexual, etc.

These terms, while certainly not exhaustive, provide a foundation for understanding and connecting with LGBTQ+ patients and for providing culturally and socially competent care. Throughout this chapter, the term "queer" is used as an umbrella term for the larger LGBTQ+ population and the diverse identities within.

The History and Impact of Queer Trauma

The LGBTQ+ community has a long-standing history of trauma, both collectively and on individual levels, that continues to impact a broad range of health outcomes. The notion of Minority Stress Theory is critical when discussing marginalized communities. This theory is the understanding of the relationship between minority and majority values or beliefs, the differences in such values, and the resulting deep history of harm and human rights violations against these minority communities [5–7]. While the extensive history of gender and sexual diversity as well as the associated marginalization these groups have faced worldwide is beyond the scope of this chapter, it is important to recognize the intersectionality of LGBTQ+ history with Black, urban, and feminist history and theory. Intersectionality in health disparities research is the complex understanding of how multiple forms of marginalization overlap or intersect and has been described over the last several decades by critical feminist writers and civil rights activists [8]. Much of the current research on queer trauma and its subsequent healthcare impacts were drawn from similar research grounded in Black feminism as well as other work assessing the negative impacts of systemic racism and historical oppression of other marginalized communities [8].

In the book, *Trauma, Resilience, and Healthcare Promotion in LGBT Patients*, Eckstrand et al. describe how sexual orientation was first used in Western medicine in the late 1890s to categorize and later pathologize individuals [9]. The neurologist Sigmund Freud described homosexuality as "a failure to fully sexually mature…an accidental deviation from normal development," including homosexuality in the same category as pedophilia, fetishism, and sadism. This led to a dangerous era of "conversion therapy" or methods used to forcibly change one's sexual orientation or gender identity, often through harmful means. These methods became increasingly prominent in the mid-twentieth century and included psychoanalysis, therapy, hypnosis, aversive conditioning, lobotomies, electroconvulsive therapy, testicular implants, bladder washing with caustic solutions, rectal massage, and physical and chemical castration [9–11].

In the post-World War II decade, thousands of war veterans, especially African-American men, were dishonorably discharged and often incarcerated or hospitalized on allegations of same-sex acts [12]. Not only were these discharges and subsequent incarcerations or hospitalizations ostracizing, but also the "blue slip" dishonorable discharge alienated veterans from the governmental resources provided by the Servicemen's Readjustment Act of 1944 (also known as the GI Bill) and limited further job prospects and access to Veteran Affairs healthcare [12]. The "Lavender Scare" and persecution of gender diverse individuals in governmental work during the McCarthy-era 1950s paralleled the more widely known "Red Scare" anti-communist campaigns, normalizing the bureaucratic institutionalization of homophobia in the United States government. These examples highlight the intersectionality and further marginalization that the LGBTQ+ community faced in the mid-1900s, especially when we consider the services of the Veteran Affairs health care system.

Physical "conversion therapy" methods gave way to behavioral therapy in the 1960s, with the Diagnostic and Statistical Manual-II (DSM-II) continuing the classification of homosexuality as a deviation of normal sexual development [10]. Backed by the significant effort of queer, political, and civil rights activists, as well as in the wake of the Stonewall Riots of 1969, homosexuality was declassified as a mental health disorder in the DSM-III in 1973-74, yet replaced by "ego-dystonic homosexuality" and "sexual orientation disturbance" in later editions [6]. Today, the DSM-5 has no diagnostic criteria that pertain to sexuality [13]. Unlike homosexuality, gender diversity and transgender identification was not included in the initial DSM, and only added in the DSM-III [13].

Today, in 2023, all major medical organizations oppose discrimination of patients based on sex, sexual orientation, or gender identity, as well oppose the use of "conversion therapies" [14]. For example, the American Psychiatric Association (APA) [15] explicitly states in their 2018 Position Statement on Conversion Therapy and LGBTQ Patients:

1. APA reaffirms its recommendation that ethical practitioners refrain from attempts to change individuals' sexual orientations.
2. APA recommends that ethical practitioners respect the identities for those with diverse gender expressions.
3. APA encourages psychotherapists which affirm individuals' sexual orientations and gender identities.
4. APA encourages legislation which would prohibit the practice of "reparative" or conversion therapies that are based on the a priori assumption that diverse sexual orientations and gender identities are mentally ill [15].

While there have been advances in the realm of LGBTQ+ equality and de-stigmatization since the 1900s, there remains significant evidence that health inequities remain for all members of the LGBTQ+ population compared to non-LGBTQ+ groups that are similar in race, socioeconomic status, and education [9]. In 2012, The Center for Medicare and Medicaid Services and the Office of the National Coordinator of Health Information Technology declined to include sexual orientation and gender identity questions in meaningful use guidelines for electronic health records [16]. It was only in 2020 that the United States Supreme Court ruled to provide employment protection for citizens based on their sexual orientation and gender identity [6]. The recent 2022 National Survey on LGBTQ Young Mental Health, polling nearly 34,000 LGBTQ youth in the USA, showed that over 10% of participants reported being threatened with or undergoing "conversion therapy," despite major medical organizations' recommendations to oppose "conversion therapy" [17]. In fact, data would suggest that "conversion therapy" is a risk factor for higher rates of attempted suicide among LGBTQ+ youth [17]. It is with this brief overview that it is critical for healthcare professionals to understand the deeper history of harm and mistrust that LGBTQ+ individuals bring with them when interfacing with healthcare systems.

An Unmet Need

The literature suggests that LGBTQ+ individuals are at a higher risk of suffering from others' negative bias, discrimination, and violence than the heterosexual or cisgender population [9, 18, 19]. Emotional and physical trauma often begins at a young age, with LGBTQ+ youth reporting significantly higher numbers of adverse childhood events (ACEs) than heterosexual youth [20]. In one study, 39% of queer teens between 14 and 18 years of age reported experiencing four or more ACEs [21]. From the 2010 National Intimate Partner and Sexual Violence Survey, lesbian, gay, and bisexual respondents reported significantly higher rates of intimate partner violence than heterosexual respondents [22]. Transgender patients similarly report higher rates of intimate partner violence compared to cisgender patients [23]. The recent 2022 National Survey on LGBTQ Young Mental Health Survey demonstrated that 45% of LGBTQ+ youth seriously considered suicide in the last year, with a staggering 14% attempting suicide [17].

Fears of (and realized) discrimination persist throughout adulthood in a variety of arenas. In an international meta-analysis of 386 studies centered on non-heterosexual individuals, 55% reported verbal harassment, 45% reported sexual harassment, and 41% reported some experience of discrimination [24, 25]. Experiences of discrimination occurred on both personal and institutional levels, as many study participants resided in counties either with explicit anti-LGBTQ+ laws or where laws did not provide protection against discriminatory behavior.

Fears of stigma influence the manner in which queer people interact with the healthcare system. When LGBTQ+ people are not legally protected from harm, they report increased hesitation in accessing care [25–27]. LGBTQ+ individuals are more likely to delay or avoid seeking medical care due to fear of mistreatment and may withhold information from healthcare professionals or allow those professionals to assume a heterosexual orientation [28–32]. In a small mixed methods' study of 20 lesbian veterans within the Veterans Affairs health system, nearly half of respondents feared their healthcare professionals would mistreat them if they knew about their sexual orientation [33]. In addition, LGBTQ+ people are more likely to report overall dissatisfaction with the healthcare they receive [25, 26, 34].

Avoidance of healthcare due to experienced or feared discrimination likely contributes to the myriad health disparities affecting sexual and gender minorities. Various studies have reported higher incidence of musculoskeletal disorders, gastrointestinal and hepatic disease, renal disease, and certain types of cancer in different parts of the LGBTQ+ population [25, 35, 36]. These disparities extend to mental health as well, with queer individuals reporting a higher incidence of depression, anxiety, suicidal ideation or attempts, and substance use compared to heterosexual peers due to the traumatizing nature of homophobia, transphobia, and other abusive and/or discriminatory behaviors directed at them [37].

These data are striking and highlight the imperative for change on a large scale. Literature focused on improving LGBTQ+ health care indicates that there are many elements of the patient experience that can be modified by healthcare professionals or organizations to make a substantial impact on the wellbeing of queer individuals.

An Introduction to Trauma-Informed Care in the Reproductive Setting

Establishing an environment in which queer patients feel safe and secure is critical to building trust in the health system. Given the aforementioned history of LGBTQ+ trauma at the hands of medical professionals, many healthcare professionals have begun to employ trauma-informed care (TIC) principles in order to provide a safe and secure medical environment. TIC involves acknowledgment of an individual's past traumas or personal history and how it may affect a person's experience of health care. TIC is performed with the ethos of augmenting medical care to offer a holistic and empathetic approach to patient care. The notion of TIC was introduced in the 1990s in the psychiatric literature as a framework to provide more compassionate and sensitive care to those with post-traumatic stress disorder as mental health research demonstrated associations between trauma exposure and psychiatric conditions [6, 38]. There are many understandings and generalized definitions of TIC. The National Center for Trauma Informed Care's (NCTIC) six principles of TIC are safety, trustworthiness and transparency, peer support, collaboration and mutuality, empowerment and choice, and cultural and gender identity [39]. As described by Goodman et al., five general dimensions are [40]:

1. Fostering agency and mutual respect;
2. Providing psychoeducation;
3. Increasing opportunities to connect with other survivors;
4. Building on clients' strengths; and.
5. Practicing cultural sensitivity.

From the Substance Abuse and Mental Health Services Administration (SAMHSA), TIC includes [41]:

1. Realization of the widespread impact of trauma and understanding of potential paths for recovery,
2. Recognition of signs and symptoms of trauma;
3. Response that integrates knowledge about trauma into policies, procedures, and practices; and.
4. Prevention of re-traumatization.

Studies have shown that incorporating TIC into clinical practice improves patient outcomes, particularly in the realm of mental health. In one study where primary care healthcare professionals were randomized to receive TIC training, those healthcare professionals that received the training described an increase in patient-centeredness based on a quantitative scoring system [42]. In a large study of over 200 LGBTQ+ interpersonal violence (IPV) survivors, those who perceived greater levels of TIC had greater emotional regulation and lower degrees of social withdrawal [43]. Another study of nearly 300 LGBTQ+ IPV survivors who received TIC mental health counseling showed that when there was a greater emphasis on agency and mutual respect, patients reported lower depression symptoms [44].

TIC studies have historically focused on mental health services, with little evidence on reproductive healthcare [6]. Mental health services are critically important given the higher rates of IPV and associated detrimental mental health outcomes among the queer community [22]. Nevertheless, reproductive healthcare professionals hold a unique opportunity to provide competent and sensitive TIC for their patients. Over the last decade, there has been more research on the lasting impacts of emotional and physical trauma on reproductive health outcomes. There is evidence that a history of trauma exposure leads to worsened prenatal, intrapartum, and postpartum outcomes, such as low birth weight, preterm delivery, increased fetal death, poor maternal-infant bonding, and early cessation of breastfeeding [45–47]. Gynecologic studies demonstrate that a history of trauma is a risk factor for increased rates of chronic pelvic pain and sexual dysfunction [48, 49].

In the reproductive setting, LGBTQ+ patients often seek the services of fertility clinics for family building. Increasingly more LGBTQ+ patients are using assisted reproductive technology (ART) for genetically related children [50]. Compared to a cisgender population, a larger proportion of LGBTQ+ patients present to the fertility clinic without any infertility diagnosis [51]. Options such as reciprocal or co-IVF for same-sex female patients and high rates of gestational carriers for same-sex male patients are unique to this population. Given the reliance on the medical system for genetically related children, interactions at the fertility clinic can be inherently stressful for LGBTQ+ patients. Moreover, the frequency of clinical visits with pelvic and speculum exams and pelvic ultrasounds may deter LGBTQ+ patients who may otherwise not engage in penetrative intercourse or have genital dysphoria [52–54]. Legal protections specifically regarding reproductive care with ART for gender diverse patients differ state to state and is a complex and actively shifting legal topic that is beyond the scope of this chapter. The fertility clinic is an excellent example of a medicalized space where healthcare professionals have an opportunity to create a TIC approach to providing care for a historically marginalized community [50]. The American Society for Reproductive Medicine (ASRM) has recently published a statement that explicitly addresses that "infertility clinics should treat persons equally regardless of sexual orientation or gender identity" [55].

Importantly, TIC does not assume a universal history of trauma and can bridge into other non-trauma facets of reproductive healthcare. For example, women who have sex with women experience cervical cancer at similar rates as heterosexual women yet are significantly less likely to obtain routine Pap testing [56, 57]. A potential TIC approach to this situation may employ methods for universal screening of patients, avoiding the assumption that women who have sex with women do not develop cervical cancer.

Recommendations to Provide Trauma-Informed Care in the LGBTQ+ Reproductive Population

Given the sordid history and oftentimes current practice of medical marginalization of the LGBTQ+ population, it is medical professionals' responsibility to incorporate a trauma-informed approach to their medical practice. Medical prejudice and discriminatory practices are not inevitable and can be mitigated with education, motivation, and resources [58]. TIC may not seem any different from the usual provision of good clinical care, given its roots in patient autonomy, respect, cultural sensitivity, and patient empowerment [6]. Nevertheless, we know that obstetrics and gynecology trainees often feel unprepared on how to screen and address trauma [39, 59]. In another survey of obstetrician gynecologists, only 29% of respondents reported that they felt comfortable caring for transgender patients, and 11% were unwilling to perform screening Pap tests [60, 61].

There are many ways to perform competent and compassionate TIC in the reproductive setting. Before patients even reach a clinic, healthcare professionals should advocate for a change in the work culture, hire trauma-competent staff, and offer training sessions for all staff [6, 38, 61]. Infrastructure including visible signs of representation in the waiting room and gender-neutral restrooms are ways to show that patients of all backgrounds, relationships, and genders are welcomed and safe [6].

When interacting with patients, a core component of TIC is to establish the patient as the expert in their own life and experience [6]. Being sensitive to, and inclusive of, the labels people use to characterize their identity can help assure patients of a respectful environment. To promote inclusivity and avoid errors of language, all patients should be asked about their preferences for names and pronouns. Additionally, attempts to avoid gendered honorifics, such as "Ms." or "Mr.", should always be made [61]. Healthcare professionals can also implement a non-gendered protocol for calling patients for an appointment, for example by simply using first names or initials—"Matthew S." as opposed to "Mr. Smith." Healthcare professionals can further normalize these topics by offering their own pronouns during introductions.

Attention should be paid to the language used in all signage, documentation, and in-person interactions. In a mixed methods study of over 200 nurses about LGBTQ+ knowledge and inclusivity, only 5% of agencies used gender inclusive forms, 44% of nurses did not know what "gender inclusive" meant, and 14% of nurses confused gender with sexual orientation [62]. Staff knowledge of appropriate terminology surrounding gender and sexual orientation should be assessed in a non-judgmental way, with education provided as needed. Intake forms should include a range of genders, sexual orientations, and other ways for patients to safely share their unique identity with their healthcare teams [6, 62]. Medical forms should ideally have a free-response format as opposed to multiple choice. For example, allowing patients to simply note their gender identity recognizes a much broader range of human experience than having to simply circle "man, woman, or other." When appropriate, patients should receive LGBTQ-specific patient education materials that avoid gendered terms and assumptions about patient experiences [32].

The issue of language is especially prominent in reproductive healthcare, as many hospitals, clinics, or services continue to be labeled with gendered names, such as "women's hospital," "men's health," or "well woman exam." These names are the result of outdated assumptions stemming from the gender/sex binary. For example, society recognizes that not all cisgender women can become pregnant due to a variety of reasons, but fails to recognize that others besides women, such as transgender men or some non-binary individuals, can carry a pregnancy. A more inclusive, culturally competent approach is to avoid gendered language and simply refer objectively to anatomy or physiology. The American Journal of Obstetrics and Gynecology published a Call to Action in 2018 regarding the use of gender inclusive language [63]. Some examples include:

1. Re-labeling "women's health clinics" as "sexual and reproductive health services".

2. Using the term "pregnant individuals" as opposed to terms such as "expectant mothers".
3. Designating the purpose of visits as "cervical cancer screening" as opposed to a "well woman exam."

Along with the avoidance of gendered language, healthcare professionals should also avoid making assumptions regarding what anatomy a patient has, what types of sexual activities they might engage in, or which health screenings they require based on their name, pronouns, or appearance [63]. In order to guide appropriate care, healthcare professionals should ask objective, clarifying questions. Examples include, "do you have a uterus/cervix?" or "do you have oral/anal sex?" Importantly, these questions should be directly related to the care being provided, and the patient should understand the medical rationale for asking these questions. In the case of fertility care or the care of couples, it is important to avoid assumptions regarding family or relational structure. In the case of a partnered couple expecting a child, there is not always a "mother" and a "father." Similarly, for fertility care, we recommend using open-ended questions regarding the intended source of sperm, source of an egg, and who will carry the pregnancy.

It is critical to take a trauma-informed approach to physical exams, as many visits for sexual or reproductive health involve invasive exams that can be uncomfortable or even directly triggering for patients. Intimate partner violence or interpersonal violence (IPV) is physical, sexual, psychological, or emotional violence from a current or former partner [64, 65]. A history of IPV is an important risk factor for PTSD and chronic pelvic pain [66], and genital exams have the potential to elicit flashbacks and increase levels of anxiety in up to 50% of people who have experienced sexual assault [67]. Additionally, data suggest that LGBTQ+ individuals are more likely to experience IPV compared to the cisgender, heterosexual population. In one nationally representative survey, the United States Centers for Disease Control and Prevention (CDC) noted that among the cisgender population, 44% of lesbian women, 61% of bisexual women, and 63% of gay or bisexual men reported IPV, compared with 29% of heterosexual men and 35% of heterosexual women [22]. Furthermore, the issue of IPV may be even more pronounced in the transgender population. A systematic review and meta-analysis including data from 49,996 transgender individuals reported a median lifetime prevalence of physical IPV of 37.5%, sexual IPV 25%, physical IPV in the past year 16.7%, and sexual IPV in the last year 10.8% [64, 65]. Compared with cisgender individuals, transgender individuals were more likely to experience any kind of IPV with a relative risk (RR) of 1.7 for any IPV, RR 2.2 for physical IPV, and RR 2.5 for sexual IPV [64, 65]. Additionally, LGBTQ+ individuals have a greater risk of sexual assault, with transgender individuals having the greatest risk [19].

Pelvic exams—truly, any physical exams—should always be performed with sensitivity and respect. Given the high prevalence of IPV and sexual assault among the LGBTQ+ population, these principles are even more important. It is critical to acknowledge the power dynamic between the healthcare professional, who possesses knowledge and controls access to desired or needed healthcare, and the patient who is inherently in a vulnerable position [64, 65]. The following recommendations are aimed at transitioning power from the healthcare professional to the patient:

1. Ask for and use patients' pronouns and desired name as well as patient preference for names of body parts and medical examinations?
2. Clearly explain the medical rationale for any physical examination, as well as what to expect before, during, and after the examination.
3. Allow the patient to manage the setting and performance of the examination to the greatest extent feasible. Below are several examples that promote patient empowerment and agency:

    (a) Consider the timing of the exam: Some patients may wish to get to know healthcare professionals on an initial encounter and return at a later date for an examination.
    (b) If desired, allow the patient the opportunity to have their desired support person present. We recommend, as supported by the American College of Obstetricians and Gynecologists (ACOG), always having a chaperone present during sensitive examinations for both healthcare professional and patient protection (ACOG Committee Opinion 796) [68].
    (c) Openly discuss any questions, concerns, fears, or apprehensions the patient may have surrounding the exam or their care in general as well as possible accommodations to meet their needs.
    (d) As much of the discussion as possible should occur prior to the exam with the patient fully dressed. The healthcare professional should leave the room to allow for privacy in undressing. Likewise, individuals should be allowed to redress after the exam prior to continuing the visit.
    (e) Consider alternative solutions for patient positioning. For example, allowing the patient to shift into a "butterfly" position for a pap smear rather than utilizing footrests if desired.

4. Form a partnership. The physical exam should be performed "with" the patient, rather than "on the patient."

    (a) Healthcare professionals can consider offering a mirror to allow the patient to visualize and understand what the examiner is seeing.
    (b) Ask for consent prior to every step of the exam and walk the patient through each portion.
    (c) Patients may have a desire to place instruments themselves or self-collect swabs.
    (d) Ask patients how they are feeling emotionally and physically after the exam is completed.

While these examples are not an exhaustive list of ways to provide sensitive and competent TIC to LGBTQ+ patients in the reproductive setting, our current health inequities are solemn reminders that healthcare professionals must start somewhere. Given the history of medical marginalization, the onus is on the healthcare system and healthcare professionals to educate themselves and create the necessary change both at the individual and institutional levels.

References

1. Jones JM. U.S. LGBT identification at steady at 7.2%. Gallup. Published February 22, 2023. https://news.gallup.com/poll/470708/lgbt-identification-steady.aspx. Accessed 10 May 2023.
2. Herman JL, Flores AR, O'Neill KK. How many adults and youth identify as transgender in the United States? The Williams Institute, UCLA School of Law. 2022. Website: https://williamsinstitute.law.ucla.edu/publications/trans-adults-united-states/. Accessed 10 May 2023.
3. The World Health Organization. Gender and health. 2023. https://www.who.int/health-topics/gender#tab=tab_1. Accessed 10 May 2023.
4. Trans Student Educational Resources. Gender unicorn. 2015. https://transstudent.org/gender/. Accessed 10 May 2023.
5. Dentato MP. The minority stress perspective. Psychology and AIDS Exchange Newsletter. April 1, 2012. https://www.apa.org/pi/aids/resources/exchange/2012/04/minority-stress. Accessed 12 May 2023.
6. Levenson JS, Craig SL, Austin A. Trauma-informed and affirmative mental health practices with LGBTQ+ clients. Psychol Serv. 2023;20:134–44. https://doi.org/10.1037/ser0000540.
7. Meyer IH. Prejudice, social stress, and mental health in lesbian, gay, and bisexual populations: conceptual issues and research evidence. Psychol Bull. 2003;129:674–97. https://doi.org/10.1037/0033-2909.129.5.674.
8. Doetsch-Kidder S, Harris K. Healing justice as intersectional feminist praxis: Well-being practices for inclusion and liberation. J Int Women's Stud. 2023;25:1–18. Available at: https://vc.bridgew.edu/jiws/vol25/iss1/4
9. Eckstrand KL, Potter JS. Trauma, resilience, and health promotion in LGBT patients: what every healthcare provider should know, vol. 2017. Springer International Publishing; 2017. https://doi.org/10.1007/978-3-319-54509-7.
10. Graham TC. Conversion therapy: a brief reflection on the history of the practice and contemporary regulatory efforts. Creighton Law Rev. 2019;52:419–25. ISSN: 0011-1155
11. American Medical Association. Health Care Needs of Lesbian, Gay, Bisexual, Transgender and Queer Populations H-160.991. 2018. Retrieved from: https://policysearch.ama-ssn.org/policyfinder/detail/gender%20identity?uri=%2FAMADoc%2FHOD.xml-0-805.xml.
12. Jones JD. "To stand upon my constitutional rights": the NAACP and world war II—era esxual exclusion. J Civil Human Rights. 2016;2:121–50. https://doi.org/10.5406/jcivihumarigh.2.2.0121.
13. Robles R, Real T, Reed G. Depathologizing sexual orientation and transgender identities in psychiatric classifications. Consortium Psychiatricum. 2021;2:45–53. https://doi.org/10.17816/CP61.
14. American Medical Association. Sexual orientation and gender identity change efforts (so-called "conversion therapy"). 2022. Website: https://www.ama-assn.org/system/files/conversion-therapy-issue-brief.pdf. Accessed 10 May 2023.
15. American Psychiatric Association (APA). Position statement on conversion therapy and LGBTQ patients. 2018. Website: https://www.psychiatry.org/getattachment/3d23f2f4-1497-4537-b4de-fe32fe8761bf/Position-Conversion-Therapy.pdf. Accessed 10 May 2023.
16. Cahill S, Makadon H. Sexual orientation and gender identity data collection in clinical settings and electronic health records: a key to ending LGBT health disparities. LGBT Health. 2014;1:34–41. https://doi.org/10.1089/lgbt.2013.0001.
17. The Trevor Project. 2022 National Survey on LGBTQ Mental Health. 2022. Website: https://www.thetrevorproject.org/survey-2022/assets/static/trevor01_2022survey_final.pdf. Accessed 10 May 2023.

18. Elze DE. The lives of lesbian, gay, bisexual, and transgender people: a trauma-informed and human rights perspective. In: Butler LD, Critelli FM, Carello J, editors. Trauma and human rights. Cham: Palgrave Macmillan; 2019. p. 179–206. https://doi.org/10.1007/978-3-030-16395-2_8.
19. Truman JL and Morgan RE. Violent victimization by sexual orientation and gender identity, 2017–2020. Bureau of Justice Statistics. 2022. https://bjs.ojp.gov/content/pub/pdf/vvsogi1720.pdf. Accessed 24 Nov 2023.
20. Merrick MT, Ford DC, Ports KA, Guinn AS. Prevalence of adverse childhood experiences from the 2011-2014 behavioral risk factor surveillance system in 23 states. JAMA Pediatr. 2018;172(11):1038–44. https://doi.org/10.1001/jamapediatrics.2018.2537.
21. Craig SL, Austin A, Levenson J, Leung VWY, Eaton AD, D'Souza SA. Frequencies and patterns of adverse childhood events in LGBTQ+ youth. Child Abuse Negl. 2020;107:104623. https://doi.org/10.1016/j.chiabu.2020.104623.
22. Walters ML, Chen J, Breiding MJ. The National Intimate Partner and sexual violence survey (NISVS): 2010 findings on victimization by sexual orientation. Atlanta, GA: National Center for Injury Prevention and Control, Centers for Disease Control and Prevention; 2013. https://www.cdc.gov/violenceprevention/pdf/nisvs_sofindings.pdf. Accessed 10 May 2023
23. Langenderfer-Magruder L, Whitfield DL, Walls NE, Kattari SK, Ramos D. Experiences of intimate partner violence and subsequent police reporting among lesbian, gay, bisexual, transgender, and queer adults in Colorado: comparing rates of cisgender and transgender victimization. J Interpers Violence. 2016;31:855–71. https://doi.org/10.1177/0886260514556767.
24. Katz-Wise S, Hyde J. Victimization experiences of lesbian, gay, and bisexual individuals: a meta-analysis. J Sex Res. 2012;49:142–67. https://doi.org/10.1080/00224499.2011.637247.
25. Zeeman L, Sherriff N, Browne K, McGlynn N, Mirandol M, Gios L, et al. A review of lesbian, gay, bisexual, trans and intersex (LGBTI) health and healthcare inequalities. Eur J Pub Health. 2019;29:974–80. https://doi.org/10.1093/eurpub/cky226.
26. Elliott M, Kanouse D, Burkhart M, Abel GA, Lyratzopoulos G, Beckett MK, et al. Sexual minorities in England have poorer health and worse health care experiences: a national survey. J Gen Intern Med. 2015;30:9–16. https://doi.org/10.1007/s11606-014-2905-y.
27. Whitehead J, Shaver J, Stephenson R. Outness, stigma, and primary health care utilization among rural LGBT populations. PLoS One. 2016;11:1–17. https://doi.org/10.1371/journal.pone.0146139.
28. Klitzman RL, Greenberg JD. Patterns of communication between gay and lesbian patients and their health care providers. Journal of Homosexuality. 2002;42(4):65–75. https://doi.org/10.1300/J082v42n04_04.
29. Preston DB, D'Augelli AR, Kassab CD, Cain RE, Schulze FW, Starks MT. The influence of stigma on the sexual risk behavior of rural men who have sex with men. AIDS Educ Prev. 2004;16(4):291–303. https://doi.org/10.1521/aeap.16.4.291.40401. PMID: 15342332.
30. Rajabiun S, Mallinson RK, McCoy K, Coleman S, Drainoni ML, Rebholz C, Holbert T. "Getting me back on track": the role of outreach interventions in engaging and retaining people living with HIV/AIDS in medical care. AIDS Patient Care STDS. 2007;21 Suppl 1:S20–9. https://doi.org/10.1089/apc.2007.9990. PMID: 17563286.
31. Cochran SD, Mays VM. Disclosure of sexual preference to physicians by black lesbian and bisexual women. West J Med. 1988;149(5):616–9. PMID: 3250107; PMCID: PMC1026562.
32. Wilkerson JM, Rybicki S, Barber CA, Smolenski DJ. Creating a culturally competent clinical environment for LGBT patients. J Gay Lesbian Soc Serv. 2011;23(3):376–94. https://doi.org/10.1080/10538720.2011.589254.
33. Mattocks KM, Sullivan JC, Bertrand C, Kinney RL, Sherman MD, Gustason C. Perceived Stigma, Discrimination, and Disclosure of Sexual Orientation Among a Sample of Lesbian Veterans Receiving Care in the Department of Veterans Affairs. LGBT Health. 2015;2(2):147–53. https://doi.org/10.1089/lgbt.2014.0131.
34. Pennant M, Bayliss S, Meads C. Improving lesbian, gay and bisexual healthcare: a systematic review of qualitative literature from the UK. Divers. Health Care. 2009;6:193–203. ISSN: 2049-5471

35. Boehmer U, Ozonoff A, Miao X. An ecological analysis of colorectal cancer incidence and mortality: differences by sexual orientation. BMC Cancer. 2011;400:111–8. https://doi.org/10.1186/1471-2407-11-400.
36. Meads C, Carmona C, Kelly MP. Lesbian, gay and bisexual people's health in the UK: a theoretical critique and systematic review. Divers Equal Health Care. 2012;9:19–32.
37. King M, Semleyn J, Tai SS, Killaspy H, Osborn D, Popelyuk D, et al. A systematic review of mental disorder, suicide and deliberate self-harm in lesbian, gay and bisexual people. BMJ Psychiatry. 2008;8:1–17. https://doi.org/10.1186/1471-244X-8-70.
38. Sperlich M, Seng JS, Li Y, Taylor J, Bradbury-Jones C. Integrating trauma-informed care into maternity care practice: conceptual and practical issues. J Midwifery Womens Health. 2017;62:661–72. https://doi.org/10.1111/jmwh.12674.
39. Nagle-Yang S, Sachdeva J, Zhao LX, Shenai N, Shirvani N, Worley LLM, et al. Trauma-informed Care for Obstetric and Gynecologic Settings. Matern Child Health J. 2022;26:2362–9. https://doi.org/10.1007/s10995-022-03518-y.
40. Goodman LA, Sullivan CM, Serrata J, Perilla J, Wilson JM, Fauci JE, et al. Development and validation of the trauma informed practice scales. J Community Psychol. 2016;44:747–64. https://doi.org/10.1002/jcop.21799.
41. Mental Health Services Administration. Trauma-informed care in behavioral health services. Substance Abuse and Mental Health Services Administration. 2014. https://store.samhsa.gov/product/TIP-57-Trauma-Informed-Care-in-Behavioral-Health-Services/SMA14-4816. Accessed 10 May 2023.
42. Green BL, Saunder PA, Power E, Dass-Brailsford PD, Schelbert KB, Giller E, et al. Trauma-informed medical care: a CME communication training for primary care providers. Fam Med. 2015;47:7–14. PMID: 25646872
43. Scheer JR, Poteat VP. Trauma-informed care and health among LGBTQ intimate partner violence survivors. J Interpers Violence. 2021;36:6670–92. https://doi.org/10.1177/0886260518820688.
44. Antebi-Gruszka N, Scheer JR. Associations between trauma-informed care components and multiple health and psychosocial risks among LGBTQ survivors of intimate partner violence. J Ment Health Couns. 2021;43:139–56. https://doi.org/10.17744/mehc.43.2.04.
45. Jasthi DL, Nagle-Yang S, Frank S, Masotya M, Huth-Bocks A. Associations between adverse childhood experiences and prenatal mental health and substance use among urban, low-income women. Community Ment Health J. 2022;58:595–605. https://doi.org/10.1007/s10597-021-00862-1.
46. Meltzer-Brody S, Bledsoe-Mansori SE, Johnson N, Killian C, Hamer RM, Jackson C, et al. A prospective study of perinatal depression and trauma history in pregnant minority adolescents. Am J Obstet Gynecol. 2013;208(211):e1–7. https://doi.org/10.1016/j.ajog.2012.12.020.
47. Pastor-Moreno G, Ruiz-Pérez I, Henares-Montiel J, Petrova D. Intimate partner violence during pregnancy and risk of fetal and neonatal death: a meta-analysis with socioeconomic context indicators. Am J Obstet Gynecol. 2020, 222:123–133.e5. https://doi.org/10.1016/j.ajog.2019.07.045.
48. Basson R, Gilks T. Women's sexual dysfunction associated with psychiatric disorders and their treatment. Womens Health. 2018;14:1745506518762664. https://doi.org/10.1177/1745506518762664.
49. Krantz TE, Andrews N, Petersen TR, Dunivan GC, Montoya M, Swanson N, et al. Adverse childhood experiences among gynecology patients with chronic pelvic pain. Obstet Gynecol. 2019;134(5):1087–95. https://doi.org/10.1097/AOG.0000000000003533.
50. Raja NS, Russell CB, Moravek MB. Assisted reproductive technology: considerations for the nonheterosexual population and single parents. Fertil Steril. 2022;118(1):47–53. https://doi.org/10.1016/j.fertnstert.2022.04.012.
51. Ross LE, Tarasoff LA, Anderson S, Epstein R, Marvel S, Steele LS, Green D. Sexual and gender minority peoples' recommendations for assisted human reproduction services. J Obstet Gynaecol Can. 2014;36:146–53. https://doi.org/10.1016/S1701-2163(15)30661-7.

52. Brik T, Vrouenraets L, See S, Meissner A, de Vries MC, Hannema SE. Use of fertility preservation among a cohort of transgirls in The Netherlands. J Adolesc Health. 2019;64:589–93. https://doi.org/10.1016/j.jadohealth.2018.11.008.
53. Cheng PJ, Pastuszak AW, Myers JB, Goodwin IA, Hotaling JM. Fertility concerns of the transgender patient. Transl Androl Urol. 2019;8:209–18. https://doi.org/10.21037/tau.2019.05.09.
54. Goetsch MF, Ribbink PJA. Penetrative genital pain in transgender men using testosterone: a survey study. AJOG. 2022;226:264–70. https://doi.org/10.1016/j.ajog.2021.09.019.
55. American Society of Reproductive Medicine (ASRM) Access to fertility treatment irrespective of marital status, sexual orientation, or gender identity: an ethics committee opinion. 2021. Website: https://www.asrm.org/practice-guidance/ethics-opinions/access-to-fertility-treatment-irrespective-of-marital-status-sexual-orientation-or-gender-identity-an-ethics-committee-opinion-2021/. Accessed 24 Nov 2023.
56. Kerker BD, Mostashari F, Thorpe L. Health care access and utilization among women who have sex with women: sexual behavior and identity. J Urban Health. 2006;83:970–9. https://doi.org/10.1007/s11524-006-9096-8.
57. Valanis BG, Bowen DJ, Bassford T, Whitlock E, Charney P, Carter RA. Sexual orientation and health: comparisons in the Women's Health Initiative sample. Arch Fam Med. 2000;9:843–53. https://doi.org/10.1001/archfami.9.9.843.
58. Dovidio JF, Fiske ST. Under the radar: how unexamined biases in decision-making processes in clinical interactions can contribute to health care disparities. Am J Public Health. 2012;102:945–52. https://doi.org/10.2105/AJPH.2011.300601.
59. Unger CA. Care of the transgender patient: a survey of gynecologists' current knowledge and practice. J Womens Health (Larchmt). 2015;24(2):114–8. https://doi.org/10.1089/jwh.2014.4918. Epub 2014 Dec 19. PMID: 25525682.
60. LaPlante LM, Gopalan P, Glance J. Addressing intimate partner violence: reducing barriers and improving residents' attitudes, knowledge, and practices. Acad Psychiatry. 2016;40:825–8. https://doi.org/10.1007/s40596-016-0529-8.
61. Potter J, Peitzmeier S, Reisner S, Bernstein I. If you have it, check it: overcoming barriers to cervical cancer screening with patients on the female-to-male transgender spectrum. 2016. http://www.lgbthealtheducation.org/training/on-demand-webinars/2014. https://www.lgbtqiahealtheducation.org/courses/if-you-have-it-check-it-overcoming-barriers-to-cervical-cancer-screening-with-patients-on-the-female-to-male-transgender-spectrum/
62. Carabez R, Pellegrini M, Mankovitz A, Eliason M, Scott M. Does your organization use gender inclusive forms? Nurses' confusion about trans* terminology. J Clin Nurs. 2015;24:3306–17. https://doi.org/10.1111/jocn.12942.
63. Stroumsa D, Wu JP. Welcoming transgender and nonbinary patients: expanding the language of "women's health". Am J Obstet Gynecol. 2018;219(6):585.e1-5. https://doi.org/10.1016/j.ajog.2018.09.018.
64. Peitzmeier SM, Bernstein ID, McDowell MJ, Pardee DJ, Agénor M, Alizaga NM, Reisner SL, Potter J. Enacting power and constructing gender in cervical cancer screening encounters between transmasculine patients and health care providers. Cult Health Sex. 2020a;22(12):1315–32. https://doi.org/10.1080/13691058.2019.1677942.
65. Peitzmeier SM, Malik M, Kattari SK, Marrow E, Stephenson R, Agénor M, Reisner SL. Intimate partner violence in transgender populations: systematic review and meta-analysis of prevalence and correlates. Am J Public Health. 2020b;110(9):e1–14. https://doi.org/10.2105/AJPH.2020.305774.
66. Lampe A, Sölder E, Ennemoser A, Schubert C, Rumpold G, Söllner W. Chronic pelvic pain and previous sexual abuse. Obstet Gynecol. 2000;96(6):929–33. https://doi.org/10.1016/s0029-7844(00)01072-3.
67. Gorfinkel I, Perlow E, Macdonald S. The trauma-informed genital and gynecologic examination. CMAJ. 2021;193(23):E1090. https://doi.org/10.1503/cmaj.210331.
68. American College of Obstetricians and Gynecologists (ACOG). Committee opinion no 796: sexual misconduct. Obstet Gynecol. 2020;135:e43–50. https://doi.org/10.1097/AOG.0000000000003608.

Chapter 6
Trauma-Informed Care for Patients Who Have Experienced Racial Trauma or Discrimination

Danielle A. Kaplan

Introduction

Vanessa is a 32-year-old single Black woman employed as an attorney. Her decision to attend law school was prompted by the killing of Michael Brown, a Black teenager in Ferguson, MO, who was shot by a white police officer when he was the same age as Vanessa's youngest brother. At work, Vanessa is often mistaken for a paralegal by the older associates at the firm and she has had difficulty getting work in her practice areas of interest. When she addresses this with the mentor assigned to her by her firm, she is advised not to "cut in line."

For the last 4 years, Vanessa's menstrual cycle has been irregular. When she mentions this to her gynecologist, she is told that this is likely due to job stress and that she should have no trouble conceiving when she's ready because "your mother was extremely fertile." Although Vanessa asks if testing is necessary to determine the cause of her atypical menstrual cycle, her GYN writes her a prescription for oral contraceptives and tells her to follow up in a year.

On her own initiative, Vanessa schedules a consultation with a reproductive endocrinologist (RE), who diagnoses her with Primary Ovarian Insufficiency. He indicates that her best chance of having a child with her own gametes is to attempt to conceive now using donor sperm, and states that "IVF would be more effective but it's way more expensive so you'll probably want to do IUI".

Upset by the diagnosis and taken aback by the idea of attempting to conceive now, Vanessa begins to ask the RE a list of questions about the process. Noting that she is quite emotional, the RE tells Vanessa that her questions are best answered by the practice coordinator for the clinic's donor program and brings their

D. A. Kaplan (✉)
Department of Psychiatry, NYU-Grossman School of Medicine, New York, NY, USA
e-mail: Danielle.Kaplan@nyulangone.org

A. Lawson, A. Swanson (eds.), *Trauma-Informed Reproductive Healthcare*,
https://doi.org/10.1007/978-3-031-67474-7_6

consultation to a close. The donor program coordinator provides Vanessa with the clinic's standard orientation materials but is unable to answer questions about sperm banks with a large number of donors of color or provide her with information about support groups for infertility patients of color or Black single mothers by choice.

Vanessa decides to transfer her care to another clinic and requests a copy of her records. When she reads them, she sees that she has been described as "demanding and impatient" by her care professionals.

Like many words associated with the hot-button issues of the time, "race" and "ethnicity" are terms that are widely used and for which we lack an agreed-upon definition. Neither term accounts for the wide within-group variability that exists within any putative racial or ethnic category or acknowledges the overwhelming biological and genetic similarity that exists among groups. Those who are seen as belonging to one group in a particular cultural context might be described with a different identifier in another. For example, some estimates suggest that there are over 50 distinct ethnic groups in China, each with its own language, culture, religious observance, and geographic origins. Should members of any of these ethnic groups emigrate from China, where they might identify as Han, Zhuang, Uyghur, or Mongolian, to the USA, they would likely be identified as either "Chinese" or "Asian" [1]. Similarly, in a 2013 survey, inhabitants of Brazil used 136 distinct categories to describe the color of their skin [2]; in the USA, these categories might be collapsed into "Black," "White," or "Hispanic/Latino," none of which might have personal relevance to the people whom they purport to describe.

The existence of race and ethnicity as categories with essential meaning is questionable at best and harmful at worst. How, then, do we reconcile the fact that these categories lack specificity and consistency with the fact that membership in specific racial or ethnic groups carries such clear identity markers, consequences, and meaning for the people who belong to them?

According to Flanigan [3]:

> Race and ethnicity are social constructs, without scientific or biological meaning. The indistinct construct of racial and ethnic categories has been increasingly acknowledged, and concerns about use of these terms in medical and health research, education, and practice have been progressively recognized…The reporting of race and ethnicity should not be considered in isolation but should be accompanied by reporting of other sociodemographic factors and social determinants, including concerns about racism, disparities, and inequities, and the intersectionality of race and ethnicity with these other factors.

It is these factors—in other words, the *racialization* of groups identified as minorities rather than race itself—that form the basis for racial trauma. Although identifiers commonly used to describe racialized or minoritized groups (for example, Black, Brown, or Hispanic/Latino) will be used throughout this chapter, it is important to recall that it is the lived experience of being identified as belonging to a particular group, including systemic racism, inequities in health care, and differences in economic, geographic, and educational opportunities, that influence outcomes for people of color.

Minority Status as a Predictor of Traumatic Events

Specific estimates of trauma in minoritized populations are variable. There is some evidence to suggest that, although rates of traumatic exposure do not differ substantially among racial and ethnic groups, the types of trauma to which people are exposed might vary by minority and immigration status. For example, Black and Hispanic adolescents are more likely to report polyvictimization (i.e., exposure to more than one traumatic event) than are white adolescents [4]. Holding multiple minoritized identities (for example, being Black and transgender), also increases the risk of traumatic exposure.

Members of some minoritized groups may be at increased risk for trauma related to immigration, depending on the reason for their departure from their countries of origin and their route of entry into the USA. In one study of Latino immigrant adolescents and their caregivers, 29% of foreign-born adolescents and 34% of their parents experienced at least one traumatic event, including being robbed or physically assaulted, during their migration experience. Notably, a substantial number of participants in the study also reported that traumatic events in their country of origin, such as natural disasters or being the victim of gang violence, had prompted their decision to emigrate. Upon arrival in the USA, many families then faced conditions, such as legal, financial, and housing instability, that increased their risk of subsequent trauma exposure in the year following their arrival [5].

In contrast to the single-incident traumas discussed above, *complex trauma* is characterized by early and repeated exposure to traumatic circumstances and events. It is only recently that researchers have begun to study complex trauma exposure as it relates to minority status. However, there is a growing body of evidence that being a member of an identified racial or ethnic minority group carries an increased risk of some types of complex trauma exposure in childhood.

In a study of adverse childhood events (ACEs) as measured by the National Study of Child Health, white children had a higher likelihood of experiencing either no ACEs or a lower total number of ACEs than did their Black and Latinx counterparts. With the exception of parental mental illness and substance abuse, the risk of experiencing any individual ACE was higher for Black and Latinx children than for their white peers. Minoritized children were significantly more likely than white children to have experienced the loss of a parent through death or incarceration, witnessed or been the victim of neighborhood violence, or been treated unfairly as a result of their race [6, 7].

There is increasing support for the recognition of race-based traumatic stress as a distinct category. This framing acknowledges that the impact of racially discriminatory experiences accumulates to produce a distinct cluster of physiological and psychological sequelae. Threats of harm or injury, experiencing shameful or humiliating events related to race, and witnessing harm to other people of color in person or in the media can result in PTSD-like symptoms including hypervigilance to threat, somatic symptoms, avoidance, suspiciousness, and nightmares [8]. Race-based traumatic stress involves the risk of ongoing exposure to experiences of discrimination, microaggressions, and victimization and pervades the experiences of people of color across institutional, systemic, local, educational, and economic spheres. The impact of this chronic exposure is akin to that experienced by complex trauma survivors and has caused some researchers to propose Complex Racial Trauma (CoRT) as a distinct category of experience [9]. The frequency and pervasiveness of these experiences for people of color have caused trauma researchers to call for racism to be recognized as a public health crisis.

Furthermore, the accretion of race-based traumatic events is a risk factor for the development of PTSD in minoritized groups. Patients seen within 2 weeks of an ER visit for treatment of an acute injury were significantly more likely to experience symptoms of posttraumatic stress if they endorsed having experienced prior experiences of racial discrimination [10]. During the early months of the COVID-19 pandemic, when anti-Asian sentiment and hate crimes increased markedly, close to 70% of young Asian and Asian-American adults surveyed indicated that they or their family experienced discrimination. Approximately, 15% reported being the victims of verbal or physical assaults. These experiences were significantly related to the presence and severity of PTSD among those surveyed, irrespective of the presence of earlier mental health conditions [11].

Racial Trauma and the Medical System

The awareness of race and ethnicity as factors in one's life experience is not limited to a single generation, but involves the collective knowledge of a people's history. This collective knowledge, sometimes referred to as historical trauma, is passed across generations and involves the knowledge and implications of how a racial, ethnic, or religious group to which one belongs has been treated over time. Ethnic genocide, pogroms, slavery, lynchings, apartheid, the Holocaust, and governmental separation of Indigenous children from their parents all represent traumatic experiences that reverberate across generations. Historical trauma is often referred to as a "soul wound" [8]. However, the injuries resulting from historical trauma can extend beyond the spiritual and contribute to mistrust of the medical system.

A full discussion of historical trauma among racialized and minoritized populations involves a lifetime of sobering study and touches almost every aspect of lived experience. Of particular relevance to this discussion, however, are the ways in which the medical system has been a source of trauma for patients who are Black, Indigenous, or People of Color (BIPOC) throughout their history in the USA. The experience of patients of color in medical care, including ART, has been influenced by a long history of racism as expressed in harmful stereotypes, unethical medical treatment, economic inequities, and health inequities.

The documented history of anti-Black racism in the USA began in 1619, when the first enslaved people from Africa entered the colony of Virginia to be traded to the colonists for provisions. From their arrival in the USA, these enslaved people were valued for their capacity to engage in hard physical labor and to reproduce;

fundamental to the system of slavery was the belief that the bodies of Black men and women were uniquely able to tolerate heavy physical work and harsh physical punishment [12].

Myths about the physical resilience of Black men and women under extreme conditions were not limited to the early days of slavery. In 1793, Philadelphia was ravaged by a yellow fever epidemic that by some estimates killed 10% of the local population. Benjamin Rush, a prominent physician and signer of the Declaration of Independence, believed on the basis of anecdotal evidence that the city's Black inhabitants had innate immunity to yellow fever and a "lighter disease burden" if they did contract the disease. Based on this mistaken belief, he advocated for Philadelphia's Black residents to serve as essential workers during the epidemic, paving the way for increased contagion and death in Black communities. A similar pattern emerged during the influenza pandemic of 1918, when lack of interest in accurate epidemiological study led to an underestimate of the prevalence and mortality of the disease in Black communities. This resulted in Black nurses being pressed into service in both Black and white hospitals, again increasing the risk and mortality in their home communities [13].

These early misrepresentations of the Black body as better able to withstand physical labor, disease, and punishment negatively influenced the availability and quality of healthcare for Black patients. Equally as important, however, they continue to inform and misinform the ways in which the health and capacity of Black patients are understood by both laypeople and medical professionals.

In a 2011 telephone survey of the general population, over half the people surveyed endorsed the belief that Black people's skin was thicker than that of White people. Almost 40% endorsed the belief that Black people's blood coagulates more quickly. Close to 20% believed that Black people's nerve endings are less sensitive. In a companion study conducted several years later, these patterns of inaccurate beliefs were replicated almost exactly among medical students and residents, with over 50% of medical students surveyed endorsing at least one false belief about Black patients' health and pain tolerance [14, 15].

The implications of these false beliefs for the medical care of Black patients are stark. Studies conducted over the last 10 years consistently indicate that inaccurate beliefs about the bodies and pain tolerance of patients of color lead to these patients receiving lower-quality care. Patients of color who report pain in emergency room settings routinely receive lower rates of analgesia. Among people giving birth, Black and Latina women report higher postpartum pain scores at discharge but receive lower doses of analgesics during hospitalization and are discharged with fewer prescriptions for adequate pain management. In women's health settings, Black women presenting with pelvic pain are more likely to be misdiagnosed with pelvic inflammatory disease while alternative diagnoses such as endometriosis, which might have significant implications for their fertility, are often not considered [16–20].

The use of Black and Brown bodies for medical experimentation is by now also well-known and widely documented. Enslaved people whose illnesses and injuries made them unable to engage in intense physical labor were often solicited by medical schools as subjects of medical experimentation, a practice advertised as being of interest to medical students and economic benefit to slave owners but that was not of benefit to the ill and injured patients themselves [21]. Anatomical dissection, a cornerstone of medical education beginning in the eighteenth and nineteeth centuries, relied on the steady availability of cadavers for medical student use. The cadavers were obtained by men known to anatomy professors as "resurrectionists"; to the general population they were more commonly known as grave robbers. With fewer resources to defend their cemeteries from the practice, poor, enslaved, free Black, and immigrant communities were particularly vulnerable to having their burial sites desecrated. As described by an English journalist in the 1830s, "in Baltimore the bodies of colored people exclusively are taken for dissection because the whites do not like it, and the colored people cannot resist" [21]. Well into the twentieth century, Black men in Macon County, Alabama were recruited as research participants with promises of treatment for "bad blood." These men, involuntary participants in the infamous Tuskegee Study, were allowed to sicken and die for the purpose of allowing researchers to study the natural course of untreated syphilis, a disease for which the use of penicillin as an effective first-line treatment was already well established [22].

Many medical advances in the field of women's health have also come at the expense of the bodies of women of color. The "father of gynecology," J. Marion Sims, relied on the bodies of enslaved women, loaned or sold to him by enslavers for the purposes of medical experimentation and operated on without anesthesia, to develop the techniques that form the basis for gynecological surgery [23, 24]. He-La, the cell line obtained without consent from the cancer cells of Henrietta Lacks and widely distributed to medical researchers without her family's knowledge, has been instrumental in stem cell research and in the development of medical techniques that formed the precursors of IVF [25, 26].

Lack of consent persists in the treatment of poor and minoritized women's reproductive health. For example, recent research suggests that patients with limited English proficiency, particularly those with lower levels of education, consistently demonstrate poor understanding of the reasons for and risks associated with colposcopies, which makes it impossible for them to give truly informed consent to the procedure [27].

Strikingly, the supposed hyperfertility of Black people, prized as a continuous source of forced labor at a time when slavery was legal, is directly linked to a movement toward involuntary sterilization of Black men and women during and after Reconstruction. Government-sponsored sterilization of Black women in the South, a procedure performed so frequently that it was known colloquially as a "Mississippi appendectomy" resulted in the involuntary sterilization of up to 70,000 patients. In other parts of the country, similar government-financed sterilization programs were designed to limit the reproductive capacity of Indigenous populations and the poor in Puerto Rico [28]. Today, Latina and Native American women are far more likely than non-Hispanic White women to report that sterilization kept them from achieving their desired family size. Furthermore, Black and Latina women are more likely to report that they had insufficient or misleading information about the procedure and to report a desire for the reversal of sterilization [29–31]. As recently as 2020, researchers demonstrated a consistent trend toward the counseling of women of color toward permanent contraception options [32].

Whether or not they are aware of the specific historical events that inform their differential treatment by the healthcare system, the differences in the experiences of patients of color in medical care are readily apparent. This knowledge accompanies patients into our offices and consulting rooms and may influence their expectations of their interactions with healthcare professionals or their willingness to seek and persist in treatment. In the words of one Black woman interviewed about her experiences with reproductive healthcare,

> So, one time I had gone to the hospital because I was like overt bleeding, like really, really hard, and I shouldn't have been. …I feel like nothing happened. Like, I feel like I got an $800 bill to be looked at, asked if I was assaulted, repeatedly have to tell people I wasn't assaulted, and then be like, 'Oh, OK, go home.' And after that I really just stopped going to the doctor altogether because I felt like I didn't get any kind of help at all. So, I've wanted to go to the doctor around this fertility thing for a while. …[but] I'm just not sure that I would even get any kind of help [33].

Minoritized People in Reproductive Healthcare

Among the false beliefs endorsed by both the general population and medical professionals is the hyperfertility of patients of color [14]. Like beliefs about the pain tolerance of racialized people, the belief that people of color get pregnant easily is a direct outgrowth of the system of slavery, in which Black women were valued for their reproductive capacity. The prevalence of this mistaken belief notwithstanding, outcomes are worse for minoritized people and their babies at almost every point in the reproductive life cycle.

White patients and patients of color do not differ in their desire for pregnancy and childrearing. However, their experiences with infertility and its treatment differ at almost every step in the process. In a 2021 review article on reproductive health disparities, Jackson-Bey and her colleagues document significant differences in the reproductive health of women of color across multiple domains. Black women are significantly more likely to present with fibroids, tubal factor, and uterine factor contributors to infertility, and diminished ovarian reserve at the time of fertility consultation [34].

Women of color are also less likely to pursue infertility treatment after a diagnosis of infertility. In contrast to White women, who are frequently referred for a specialized infertility workup by their physicians, Black women are five times more like to self-refer for treatment and Latina women are four times more likely to be referred to treatment by a friend or family member. A recent study suggests that Black women wait an average of 2 years before seeking fertility treatment, compared to an average delay of 1 year among White women. The reasons for this delay include insurance coverage, geographic accessibility of clinics, cultural stigma around infertility, and prior negative experiences with the healthcare system. Whatever its causes, this delay has a critical impact on success rates and the chance of achieving a live birth [35].

Among those who do seek infertility care, outcomes are overwhelmingly worse for minoritized patients. Asian, Black, Hispanic, and Native American patients are all significantly less likely to achieve a clinical pregnancy after ART than white patients. In part, this might be a reflection of the fact that Black, Latina, and Native patients are less likely than non-Hispanic White patients to undergo IVF, which is both the gold standard for infertility treatment and among the more expensive forms of fertility care when not covered by insurance. However, minoritized patients who do use IVF are less likely to achieve a clinical pregnancy [34, 35].

These disheartening trends continue even after people of color become pregnant. Black women experience higher rates of pregnancy loss between 10 and 20 weeks gestation than do members of any other racial or ethnic group. They also experience higher rates of spontaneous abortion at any point in pregnancy overall. Racial minority status is associated with higher rates of preterm birth; very preterm infants born to Black and Hispanic mothers have higher mortality rates than those born to white mothers. Tragically, up to 40% of the disparity in infant mortality may be attributed to the quality of the hospital in which parents give birth, highlighting yet again the stark disparities in the quality of medical care across socioeconomic lines [36–39].

The widely-publicized story of tennis legend Serena Williams, who suffered from a pulmonary embolism and a hematoma requiring emergency medical treatment after the birth of her daughter via emergency Cesarean section, [40] made the general public aware of what Black patients have long known: being pregnant or postpartum while Black carries significant risk to the birthing person. Women of color experience higher rates of postpartum hemorrhage, infection, antepartum anemia and blood clots, with recent studies suggesting that antepartum anemia is associated with between one in five and one in six cases of severe maternal morbidity among Black, Hispanic, Native American, Pacific Islander, and multiracial patients. Irrespective of cause, mortality rates for Black women are 2.5 times higher than for White women. In New York City, Hispanic women are more than three times as likely and Asian American and Pacific Islander women more than four times as likely to die from pregnancy-related causes than are non-Hispanic White women [41–44].

It is not only the race of the person giving birth, but of their partner, that impacts pregnancy outcomes for patients of color. Children of Black fathers experience higher rates of preterm birth, low birth weight, and NICU admissions than do children of White fathers. Similarly, children born to Hispanic fathers have significantly lower Apgar scores and require higher rates of assisted ventilation after birth [45, 46].

Patients of color who present for fertility treatment may themselves have had prior negative experiences in reproductive care. It is highly likely that they know and care about someone who has. It is incumbent on those of us from whom patients of color seek care to be aware of both the historical antecedents of the experiences of minoritized patients in medical care and our patients' possible experiences with seeking medical care themselves and to understand the impact of this knowledge and the anxiety that it engenders on patients' expectations for treatment.

Best Practices in Addressing Racial Trauma Through Trauma-Informed Care

Cultural Competence vs. Cultural Humility

Trauma-informed care is proactive rather than reactive. In recognition of the high prevalence of trauma among patients seeking infertility and reproductive health care, a number of authors have recommended that trauma-informed practice be the standard of care for all patients [47]. Although not all minoritized patients will have had the traumatic exposures described above, such "universal precautions" represent best practices in the care of a racially and culturally diverse patient population.

Early proponents of culturally-informed care exhorted practitioners to work toward cultural competence. Cultural competence presumes that healthcare professionals can become subject-matter experts on the lived experiences of patients from diverse backgrounds and ground themselves in a set of culture-specific best practices for intercultural interaction. Leaving aside for the moment the feasibility of achieving expertise in any culture, including the ones with which we identify, best practices in trauma-informed care require us to work in a spirit of collaboration rather than assumed knowledge. A more appropriate model for working with racialized patients, then, is one in which healthcare professionals adopt an attitude of cultural humility.

As described by Ranjbar, cultural humility is "characterized by principles of mutual learning and critical self-reflection, recognition of power imbalances, and the existence of implicit biases. Its practice can engender respectful partnerships and institutional accountability. In clinical care, cultural humility can serve as a guiding concept for the practice of trauma-informed care in centering and empowering patients on their journey of healing, rather than making assumptions about the patient's experience or practicing an authoritative, power-over communication style [48]."

Cultural humility requires us to challenge our assumptions and biases about what "others" are like, asking ourselves to be in the position of student rather than expert on the lived experiences of our patients. Most importantly, however, the focus from the standpoint of cultural humility is not on gathering information about others, but on reflection about how our own experiences and biases impact how we respond to those with whose care we are entrusted.

The Clinic Environment

Although cultural humility is often conceptualized as an individual effort involving direct interactions between patient and healthcare professional, trauma-informed care for racialized patients begins at the institutional level and requires institutional accountability. For example, Title VI of the Civil Rights Act requires healthcare practitioners to assume the cost of medical interpretation for clients with limited English proficiency [49]. Forms, signage, and teaching videos must be accessible to a linguistically-diverse population and patients at varying levels of education. These measures are essential for obtaining truly informed consent, a critical first step in providing trauma-informed care.

The physical environment of our offices and clinics also provides patients with information about who is welcome and whose family-building efforts we wish to promote. Clinic websites, marketing materials, and office decor that include only White patients and babies send a clear message about the population that a clinic is interested in serving. Similarly, a mental health professional whose book collection about third-party reproduction that features only White families (or, as is common, animals), risks further alienating families of color whose experience of third-party reproduction might already have been impacted by the limited availability of Black and Brown gamete donors.

Collaboration with Patients and Diverse Healthcare Professionals

Our resource and referral lists also serve as indicators of our willingness to partner with patients of color. Culturally-informed healthcare professionals should be aware of in-person and internet-based infertility support groups and websites that center the experiences of minoritized patients. Providers who make referrals to mental health professionals should make sure that their referral lists include providers of color with specialized training in infertility counseling. Resource lists should also include information about financing the full spectrum of reproductive care, such as infertility and adoption grants that are available to patients of color.

Like all trauma-informed care, care for patients who may have experienced racial trauma is collaborative. Collaborative care involves multiple opportunities for patients to ask questions, check their comprehension, and take the necessary time to weigh their options before proceeding. Healthcare professionals should take care to ensure that the treatment options that they offer are consistent with patients' cultural and religious beliefs. Healthcare professionals should offer all options for treatment and ensure that patients are aware of the costs of each without making assumptions about the patient's insurance coverage or ability to afford out of pocket care and unilaterally deciding against offering more expensive treatment options [48, 50].

Recognizing and Addressing Implicit Bias in Fertility Care

Perhaps the most important thing that healthcare professionals can do to address racial trauma among our patients is to take care not to replicate it either overtly or as a result of implicit bias. Implicit biases are automatic beliefs that we hold toward members of an identified subgroup based on some characteristic of their identity such as age, race, gender, or disability status that is unrelated to the characteristic itself. These biases exist outside our awareness, and do not necessarily correspond to the beliefs that we profess to hold.

Implicit biases arise through repeated messaging about a designated group of people. Depictions in movies and television, news coverage, and conversations at the dinner table all contribute to our attitudes and assumptions. We may hold implicit biases about any identified subgroup, including those in which we hold membership [50, 51]. Awareness of our implicit biases is critical to ensuring that our offices, clinics, and consulting rooms are spaces of safety and support rather than of retraumatization.

The impact of implicit bias is evident across myriad contexts. It leads educators to overperceive anger in the faces of Black children and adolescents, a category error that has implications for the experience of children of color in the classroom and the legal system. Implicit bias is also associated with the overdiagnosis of psychotic disorders in Black adults and ADHD in Black children despite the existence of standardized diagnostic criteria [51, 52].

On the surface, these errors in judgment may have little to do with the world of reproductive healthcare. However, educational, legal, and psychiatric histories are routinely considered in the evaluation of gamete donors and gestational carriers, and overdiagnosis may worsen the already-existing scarcity of donors and gestational carriers of color. From the patient perspective, mental health diagnoses and legal involvement may impact educational and employment opportunities that determine patients' incomes, insurance coverage, and access to care.

Healthcare professional implicit bias does not only increase barriers to entry into fertility care for patients of color; it also impacts the likelihood that they will engage in and continue with treatment even if a referral is provided. Recent studies have shown that Black women are less likely to proceed with fertility treatment after receiving a referral, are more likely to discontinue treatment prematurely, and take longer to return for subsequent treatment cycles than do White women [35].

Implicit biases operate outside conscious awareness; as such, they may not correspond to beliefs or attitudes that we believe ourselves to hold. When medical professionals are presented with evidence of their implicit biases, reactions generally range from disappointment in the contrast between their ideals and their underlying beliefs to justification for their biases and outright rejection of the evidence [53, 54]. If our implicit biases are invisible to us, however, they are readily apparent to the patients we endeavor to serve.

Implicit bias in the infertility clinic might be manifested as overtly as an overheard comment outside the consulting room door or a disparaging note in a chart. As frequently, however, implicit bias is evident in the shorter amount of time that patients of color spend in face-to-face contact with a medical professional, the medical team's use of more negative and less complex language when speaking with patients of color, and the timeliness of getting an appointment at an infertility clinic at all when the scheduler perceives the caller on the other end of the phone to be from a minoritized group [55, 56].

Because implicit bias develops through years of exposure to messages about the stereotyped group, it is difficult to ameliorate with a single intervention. However, ethical clinical practice requires us to be aware of the existence of our implicit and explicit biases and make ongoing efforts to recognize their impact on the care we provide. There is evidence that being reminded of the existence of implicit bias, the situations in which it is most likely to manifest, and which aspects of patients' presentation to attend to can lead healthcare professionals to make more accurate diagnostic judgments and modify their treatment recommendations in the moment [57].

Patient Care:

Galiatsatos and his colleagues [58] recommend that healthcare professionals use the PLACE strategy as an in-the-moment safeguard against implicit bias. Since implicit biases are more likely to be active in situations where quick judgment is required or the amygdala is activated, *pausing* allows the healthcare professional to engage in a moment of reflection and carefully consider next steps in the interaction. *Listening* to patients involves both inquiring as to whether the patient has shared all their concerns and actively checking to ensure our own comprehension of what they have told us. Listening with a culturally-responsive ear includes engaging in dialogue with patients about treatment options that are culturally or religiously consonant for them; for BIPOC patients in particular, it might include understanding their reproductive health histories not just diagnostically, but with regard to their experiences with healthcare professionals (Table 6.1).

Trauma-informed care also involves acting as *allies* for our patients. This might require us to advocate on the patient's behalf with other members of our own staff or care team or with the clinic at which our patient is receiving care. For infertility patients whose first language is not English, for example, allyship includes a clinic-wide commitment to providing and assuming the expense for interpreters.

As is best practice in all trauma-informed care, the PLACE strategy exhorts us to *collaborate* with our patients by maintaining a respectful tone and body posture and soliciting their input on the plan of care. Finally, we are asked to *empower* our patients by giving them the tools, resources, and information they require to be full

Table 6.1 The PLACE strategy for reducing implicit bias

P	Pausing	Pause before responding to reflect and consider response. Pausing helps avoid assumptions and quick judgments
L	Listening	Asking if patients have shared all of their concerns and then checking with the patient to ensure that you have fully understood the patient
A	Ally	Advocate for the patient within own clinic or other medical setting
C	Collaborate	Ask for patient input and engage in discussion when deciding on a plan of care
E	Empower	Give patients information they need to be full partners in treatment

partners in their treatment [58]. In reproductive medicine, empowering patients of color might involve providing them with information that goes beyond the list of clinic-approved egg and sperm banks to indicate which have a higher availability of donors of color and providing them with the full range of treatment options, their associated costs, and options for financing treatment.

Although the PLACE strategy is useful for countering in-the-moment reactions as they arise, addressing implicit bias involves a repeated willingness to reflect on our own reactions and challenge our assumptions. Just as biases arise from repeated exposure to media portrayals and others' opinions of members of the stereotyped group, challenging our biases involves repeated exposure to those who are unlike us in a variety of roles and contexts. There is evidence suggesting that implicit bias may be ameliorated most effectively through prolonged, reciprocal relationships with a diverse group of friends, mentors, and colleagues. It is critically important that these relationships do not place the burden of education and raising awareness on the member of the dyad who belongs to a minoritized group. However, when feedback on our biases and missteps is offered, it is incumbent on us to respond non-defensively and reflect on what we have been told [59–61].

Expanding Social Networks As the world becomes increasingly connected through virtual spaces, the opportunities to address our biases through exposure to information about others' experiences increases. The interested healthcare professional should consider following multiple social media feeds and podcasts produced by people of color, including those that are specific to their experiences with reproductive health and fertility. Although learning about the experience of one patient does not automatically provide us with information about another, becoming familiar with common themes and experiences discussed by patients of color in reproductive healthcare provides us with an additional check on our own potential snap judgments and reactions.

Self-Reflection As in all trauma-informed care, the care of racialized patients requires us to be aware of the power and privileges that we hold. Even the most collaborative of healthcare professionals operates from a position of power. Healthcare professionals in independent practice schedule appointments at their own discretion. Healthcare professionals across disciplines routinely make decisions about when to refer patients for consultations for fertility preservation or infertility evaluations. We each hold multiple identities, each of which confers different degrees of power, privilege, or oppression. Reflecting on these identities, for example, through reading lay and academic works about the experiences of groups other than our own, and acknowledging those that might be most salient to our patients can help us understand how we are perceived by the patients we wish to serve and approach patient interactions from a more collaborative and egalitarian stance [62, 63].

Advocating for Change A comprehensive trauma-informed approach to care for patients who have experienced racial trauma requires us to demand systemic and institutional accountability. Our responsibility as professionals to examine our own biases and identities coexist with the need to advocate for wider systemic change. Advocating for increased access to reproductive care, a range of affordable treatment options, broader insurance coverage for ART and affiliated services, and recruitment of diverse third-party collaborators (e.g., sperm/egg donors and gestational carriers) are all necessary to ensure that minoritized patients have the possibility of accessing the services we provide. Similarly, it is incumbent on the current generation of healthcare professionals to advocate for diversity in the academic pipeline and provide mentorship to emerging professionals of color to increase the odds of having a truly representative array of healthcare professionals for our patients. At the same time, it is incumbent on us to engage in the internal work that allows us to welcome all patients to our practices with respect, understanding, and collaboration.

All of us—infertility patients and those who care for them alike—carry our histories with us. For racialized and minoritized patients, this history involves what is at times a personal and always a multigenerational experience of misuse, misunderstanding, and mistreatment by the medical system. For healthcare professionals, regardless of their own backgrounds, it involves biases and beliefs about minoritized patients that can result in differential treatment and errors in clinical judgment when working with patients of color. Understanding this reality and working on an individual, clinic-wide, and systemic level to address the risk of resultant harm to our patients, represents a core competency for healthcare professionals across the spectrum of reproductive and infertility care and is critical in the provision of compassionate, equitable, and trauma-informed care.

References

1. Guo R. China ethnic statistical yearbook 2020. Cham: Springer Nature; 2020.
2. Travassos C, Laguardia J, Marques PM, Mota JC, Szwarcwald CL. Comparison between two race/skin color classifications in relation to health-related outcomes in Brazil. Int J Equity Health. 2011;10(1):1–8.
3. Flanagin A, Frey T, Christiansen SL, AMA Manual of Style Committee. Updated guidance on the reporting of race and ethnicity in medical and science journals. JAMA. 2021;326(7):621–7.
4. Andrews AR, López CM, Snyder A, Saunders B, Kilpatrick D. Polyvictimization, related symptoms, and familial and neighborhood contexts as longitudinal mediators of racial/ethnic disparities in violence exposure across adolescence. J Immigr Minor Health. 2019;(21):679–92.
5. Perreira KM, Ornelas I. Painful passages: traumatic experiences and post-traumatic stress among US immigrant Latino adolescents and their primary caregivers. Int Migr Rev. 2013;47(4):976–1005.
6. Maguire-Jack K, Lanier P, Lombardi B. Investigating racial differences in clusters of adverse childhood experiences. Am J of Orthopsychiatry. 2020;90(1):106.
7. Sacks V, Murphey D. The prevalence of adverse childhood experiences, nationally, by state, and by race or ethnicity. 2018. https://www.childtrends.org/publications/prevalence-adverse-childhood-experiences-nationally-state-race-ethnicity. Accessed 19 May 2023.
8. Comas-Díaz L, Hall GN, Neville HA. Racial trauma: theory, research, and healing: introduction to the special issue. Am Psychol. 2019;74(1):1.
9. Cénat JM. Complex racial trauma: evidence, theory, assessment, and treatment. Perspect Psychol Sci. 2022;18(3):675–87.
10. Bird CM, Webb EK, Schramm AT, Torres L, Larson C, deRoon-Cassini TA. Racial discrimination is associated with acute posttraumatic stress symptoms and predicts future posttrau-

matic stress disorder symptom severity in trauma-exposed Black adults in the United States. J Traum Stress. 2021;34(5):995–1004.
11. Hahm HC, Ha Y, Scott JC, Wongchai V, Chen JA, Liu CH. Perceived COVID-19-related anti-Asian discrimination predicts post traumatic stress disorder symptoms among Asian and Asian American young adults. Psychiatry Res. 2021;303:114084.
12. Villarosa L. Myths about physical racial differences were used to justify slavery—and are still believed by doctors today. New York Times. 2019;1619.
13. Evans MK. Covid's color line—infectious disease, inequity, and racial justice. N Engl J Med. 2020;383(5):408–10.
14. Trawalter S, Hoffman KM. Got pain? Racial bias in perceptions of pain. Soc Pers Psychol Compass. 2015;9(3):146–57.
15. Hoffman KM, Trawalter S, Axt JR, Oliver MN. Racial bias in pain assessment and treatment recommendations, and false beliefs about biological differences between blacks and whites. Proc Natl Acad Sci U S A. 2016;113(16):4296–301.
16. Lloyd EP, Lloyd AR, McConnell AR, Hugenberg K. Race deficits in pain detection: medical providers and laypeople fail to accurately perceive pain authenticity among black people. Soc Psychol Pers Sci. 2022;13(5):895–905.
17. FitzGerald C, Hurst S. Implicit bias in healthcare professionals: a systematic review. BMC Med Ethics. 2017;18(1):1–8.
18. Badreldin N, Grobman WA, Yee LM. Racial disparities in postpartum pain management. Obstet Gynecol. 2019;134(6):1147.
19. Richard-Davis G, Morris JR. No longer separate but not close to equal: navigating inclusivity in a burgeoning field built on injustice. Fertil Steril. 2023;120(3):400–2.
20. Seth S. Reifying racism in medicine. Science. 2022;378(6619):481.
21. Halperin EC. The poor, the black, and the marginalized as the source of cadavers in United States anatomical education. Clin Anat. 2007;20(5):489–95.
22. Tobin MJ. Fiftieth anniversary of uncovering the Tuskegee syphilis study: the story and timeless lessons. Am J Respir Crit Care Med. 2022;205(10):1145–58.
23. Wailoo K. Historical aspects of race and medicine: the case of J. Marion Sims. JAMA. 2018;320(15):1529–30.
24. Cronin M. Anarcha, Betsey, Lucy, and the women whose names were not recorded: the legacy of J Marion Sims. Anaesth Intensive Care. 2020;48(3_suppl):6–13.
25. Skloot R. The immortal life of Henrietta Lacks. New York: Random House/Broadway Books; 2011.
26. Baptiste DL, Caviness-Ashe N, Josiah N, Commodore-Mensah Y, Arscott J, Wilson PR, Starks S. Henrietta Lacks and America's dark history of research involving African Americans. Nurs Open. 2022;9(5):2236–8.
27. Krankl JT, Shaykevich S, Lipsitz S, Lehmann LS. Patient predictors of colposcopy comprehension of consent among English-and Spanish-speaking women. Womens Health Issues. 2011;21(1):80–5.
28. Kozhimannil KB, Hassan A, Hardeman RR. Abortion access as a racial justice issue. N Engl J Med. 2022;387(17):1537–9.
29. Shreffler KM, McQuillan J, Greil AL, Johnson DR. Surgical sterilization, regret, and race: Contemporary patterns. Soc Sci Res. 2015;50:31–45.
30. Schickler R, Whittum M, Fanarjian N, Rapkin R, Nguyen BT. The history of female surgical sterilization: a social and ethics perspective. J Gynecol Surg. 2021;37(6):465–9.
31. Liddell JL, Herzberg J. "They didn't talk about stuff like that": sexual health education experiences of a Native American Tribe in the Gulf Coast. Am J Sex Educ. 2023;18(2):231–60.
32. Kathawa CA, Arora KS. Implicit bias in counseling for permanent contraception: historical context and recommendations for counseling. Health Equity. 2020;4(1):326–9.
33. Thompson TA, Young YY, Bass TM, Baker S, Njoku O, Norwood J, Simpson M. Racism runs through it: examining the sexual and reproductive health experience of Black women in the South: study examines the sexual and reproductive health experiences of Black women in the South. Health Aff. 2022;41(2):195–202.

34. Jackson-Bey T, Morris J, Jasper E, Edwards DR, Thornton K, Richard-Davis G, Plowden TC. Systematic review of racial and ethnic disparities in reproductive endocrinology and infertility: where do we stand today? F&S Rev. 2021;2(3):169–88.
35. Weiss MS, Marsh EE. Navigating unequal paths: racial disparities in the infertility journey. Obstet Gynecol. 2023;142(4):940–7. https://doi.org/10.1097/AOG.0000000000005354.
36. Mukherjee S, Velez Edwards DR, Baird DD, Savitz DA, Hartmann KE. Risk of miscarriage among black women and white women in a US prospective cohort study. Am J Epidemiol. 2013;177(11):1271–8.
37. Zore T. How your race or ethnicity may impact fertility. 2022. https://ro.co/health-guide/race-ethnicity-fertility/. Accessed 15 May 2023.
38. Oliver-Williams CT, Steer PJ. Racial variation in the number of spontaneous abortions before a first successful pregnancy, and effects on subsequent pregnancies. Int J Gynaecol Obstet. 2015;129(3):207–12.
39. Howell EA, Janevic T, Hebert PL, Egorova NN, Balbierz A, Zeitlin J. Differences in morbidity and mortality rates in black, white, and Hispanic very preterm infants among New York City hospitals. JAMA Pediatr. 2018;172(3):269–77.
40. Williams S. What my life-threatening experience taught me about giving birth. 2018. https://www.cnn.com/2018/02/20/opinions/protect-mother-pregnancy-williams-opinion/index.html. Accessed 17 May 2023.
41. Krenitsky N, Friedman AM, Yu K, Gyamfi-Bannerman C, Williams-Kane J, O'Shaugnessy F, Huang Y, Wright JD, D'Alton ME, Wen T. Trends in venous thromboembolism and associated risk factors during delivery hospitalizations from 2000 to 2018. Obstet Gynecol. 2022;139(2):223–34.
42. Igbinosa II, Leonard SA, Noelette F, Davies-Balch S, Carmichael SL, Main E, Lyell DJ. Racial and ethnic disparities in anemia and severe maternal morbidity. Obstet Gynecol. 2023;142(4):845–54. https://doi.org/10.1097/AOG.0000000000005325.
43. Hoyert DL, Miniño AM. Maternal mortality in the United States: changes in coding, publication, and data release, 2018. Natl Vital Stat Rep. 2020;69(2):1–18.
44. MacDorman MF, Thoma M, Declcerq E, Howell EA. Racial and ethnic disparities in maternal mortality in the United States using enhanced vital records, 2016–2017. Am J Public Health. 2021;111(9):1673–81.
45. Palatnik A, Garacci E, Walker RJ, Ozieh MN, Williams JS, Egede LE. The association of paternal race and ethnicity with adverse pregnancy outcomes in a contemporary US Cohort. Am J Perinatol. 2021;38(07):698–706.
46. Payne-Sturges DC, Puett R, Cory-Slechta DA. Both parents matter: a national-scale analysis of parental race/ethnicity, disparities in prenatal PM2. 5 exposures and related impacts on birth outcomes. Environ Health. 2022;21(1):47.
47. Owens L, Terrell S, Low LK, Loder C, Rhizal D, Scheiman L, Seng J. Universal precautions: the case for consistently trauma-informed reproductive healthcare. Am J Obstet Gynecol. 2022;226(5):671–7.
48. Ranjbar N, Erb M, Mohammad O, Moreno FA. Trauma-informed care and cultural humility in the mental health care of people from minoritized communities. Focus. 2020;18(1):8–15.
49. Le Neveu M, Berger Z, Gross M. Lost in translation: the role of interpreters on labor and delivery. Health Equity. 2020;4(1):406–9.
50. Greenwald AG, Dasgupta N, Dovidio JF, Kang J, Moss-Racusin CA, Teachman BA. Implicit-bias remedies: treating discriminatory bias as a public-health problem. Psychol Sci Public Interest. 2022;23(1):7–40.
51. Londono Tobon A, Flores JM, Taylor JH, Johnson I, Landeros-Weisenberger A, Aboiralor O, Avila-Quintero VJ, Bloch MH. Racial implicit associations in psychiatric diagnosis, treatment, and compliance expectations. Acad Psychiatry. 2021;45:23–33.
52. Fadus MC, Ginsburg KR, Sobowale K, Halliday-Boykins CA, Bryant BE, Gray KM, Squeglia LM. Unconscious bias and the diagnosis of disruptive behavior disorders and ADHD in African American and Hispanic youth. Acad Psychiatry. 2020;44:95–102.

53. Sukhera J, Watling CJ, Gonzalez CM. Implicit bias in health professions: from recognition to transformation. Acad Med. 2020;95(5):717–23.
54. Sukhera J, Wodzinski M, Milne A, Teunissen PW, Lingard L, Watling C. Implicit bias and the feedback paradox: exploring how health professionals engage with feedback while questioning its credibility. Acad Med. 2019;94(8):1204–10.
55. Wolsiefer KJ, Mehl M, Moskowitz GB, Cagno CK, Zestcott CA, Tejeda-Padron A, Stone J. Investigating the relationship between resident physician implicit bias and language use during a clinical encounter with Hispanic patients. Health Commun. 2023;38(1):124–32.
56. Wisniewski JM, Walker B. Association of simulated patient race/ethnicity with scheduling of primary care appointments. JAMA Netw Open. 2020;3(1):e1920010.
57. Ungar T, Knaak S, Mantler E. Making the implicit explicit: a visual model for lowering the risk of implicit bias of mental/behavioural disorders on safety and quality of care. Healthc Manage Forum. 2021;34(2):72–6. Los Angeles, CA: SAGE Publications.
58. Galiatsatos P, O'Conor KJ, Wilson C, Myers C, Reeves J, Thomas WJ, Phillips A, Johnson S, Golden SH. A checklist to address implicit bias in healthcare settings during the COVID-19 pandemic: the PLACE strategy. Health Secur. 2022;20(3):261–3.
59. Gawronski B. Six lessons for a cogent science of implicit bias and its criticism. Perspect Psychol Sci. 2019;14(4):574–95.
60. Stevens FL, Abernethy AD. Neuroscience and racism: the power of groups for overcoming implicit bias. Int J Group Psychother. 2018;68(4):561–84.
61. DiAngelo R. White fragility: why it's so hard for white people to talk about race. Boston: Beacon Press; 2018.
62. Merino Y, Adams L, Hall WJ. Implicit bias and mental health professionals: priorities and directions for research. Psychiatr Serv. 2018;69:723–5.
63. Voigt PE, Blakemore JK, McCulloh D, Fino ME. Equal opportunity for all? An analysis of race and ethnicity in fertility preservation in New York City. J Assist Reprod Genet. 2020;37:3095–102.

Chapter 7
Trauma-Informed Care: Strategies for Medical Professionals in the Reproductive Endocrinology and Infertility Clinic

Julie Bindeman and Vickie Schafer

From the time a patient calls to schedule an appointment with their fertility clinic until the time they arrive for their first appointment, negative assumptions can easily be formed by their reproductive endocrinologist and/or clinic staff that could have a long-lasting impact on the care that the patient receives. Most patients walking through a fertility clinic's doors are sad and/or anxious that they have not been able to conceive on their own, have experienced reproductive loss(es), have not yet found a partner with whom to grow their family, have been diagnosed with a life-threatening illness (e.g., cancer), and/or require third-party reproduction to grow their family. This anxiety about whether or not they will be able to be parents, will survive their illness, or will be treated in a supportive or discriminatory manner may be palpable to schedulers, the front desk team, and healthcare professionals who may mistakenly view these emotional reactions as a sign of a "difficult" patient. These early biased judgments may negatively influence interactions with patients throughout the course of their fertility treatment. To minimize potential (inadvertent) harm that can befall a patient, it is essential for practitioners and their staff to be trauma-informed. "Trauma-informed" can take on a host of definitions by healthcare professionals, many of which do not translate well to actual patient care, as they are under-representations of what it truly means to be trauma-informed and trauma-competent. Thus, this chapter focuses on the empirically supported implementation of trauma-informed care.

The study of trauma-informed care (TIC) has been centralized for many years within the field of oncology, where difficult conversations are normative with patients. In the practice of reproductive medicine, TIC should be equally centralized as infertility and reproductive loss may be perceived as equally traumatizing as

J. Bindeman (✉)
Integrative Therapy of Greater Washington, Rockville, MD, USA

V. Schafer
Private Practice, Austin, TX, USA

A. Lawson, A. Swanson (eds.), *Trauma-Informed Reproductive Healthcare*,
https://doi.org/10.1007/978-3-031-67474-7_7

cancer and as difficult conversations (e.g., pregnancy loss, negative pregnancy tests) are also a part of daily work with fertility patients [1]. Regardless of medical experience or diagnosis, it is important to view TIC as more expansive than what events might have happened to a person (i.e., stillbirth) and instead take into account the patients' backgrounds and lived experiences. Ensuring that clinics are designed to be trauma-informed, the staff is trained to be aware of potential trauma, and procedures are refashioned so that minimal trauma occurs and patients do not experience re-traumatization is equally important to the basics of knowing a patient's history and circumstances.

This chapter will apply the concepts of trauma-informed care (TIC) within the context of a reproductive endocrinology and infertility (REI) clinic. Using the Substance Abuse and Mental Health Administration's (SAMHSA) six key principles of TIC (safety; trustworthiness and transparency; peer support; collaboration and mutuality; empowerment, voice, and choice; cultural, historical, and gender issues) [2], strategies will be presented to assist clinics in adopting practices that enhance the care and satisfaction of patients while also attending to the well-being of the medical professional. Additional sections of this chapter include reviewing methods to assess for a history of trauma with patients as well as obtaining consent and its importance in TIC. Case examples and sample scripts are presented, followed by a review of methods for sharing difficult news. This chapter will conclude by reviewing strategies to reduce compassion fatigue and burnout in healthcare professionals.

Understanding the Trauma of Infertility, Fertility Preservation, and Pregnancy Loss

As discussed in prior chapters, infertility, planned and medical gamete cryopreservation, and pregnancy loss may be perceived by those who experience them as traumatic. Patients diagnosed with infertility, pregnancy loss, cancer, or who otherwise need fertility treatment to grow their families often experience a feeling of loss of control which can lead to feelings of sadness, anxiety, and grief [1, 3]. Given that many people who have experienced trauma have experienced or feared experiencing stigmatization or blame for the traumatic event (e.g., blaming rape victims for what they were wearing), those in need of fertility treatment may fear they will similarly be blamed by their reproductive endocrinology team for their condition/experiences (e.g., blaming patients' stress as the cause of infertility or loss). Given that the perception of having experienced trauma is subjective to the individual (e.g., "trauma is in the eye of the beholder") REI team members also should understand that patients may view experiences such as failed fertilization or embryos which do not make it to cryopreservation, failed embryo transfer, the identification of aneuploid embryos, negative pregnancy tests, biochemical pregnancy loss, disposition of supernumerary embryos, and other aspects of fertility treatment to be intensely distressing. Although healthcare professionals may not view these experiences as worthy of distress, in the context of TIC the healthcare professionals' beliefs are not prioritized, and it is imperative that they provide nonjudgmental emotional support for patients in distress. The provision of empathy in patient care does not mean that the healthcare professional has to agree that the experience is traumatic, instead it means the healthcare professional should empathetically try to understand why it is traumatic to the patient and provide emotional support.

Assessing for Trauma and Examination of the Role of the Healthcare Professionals' Lived Experiences

As TIC has become more widely accepted and standard in the practice of medicine, it has become increasingly clear that treating all patients from a trauma-informed perspective which recognizes the frequency of health and other consequences of trauma is beneficial. Research finds that the risk of trauma exposure is high for all individuals throughout their lives and as such, the recommendations within this chapter can and should be applied to all patients, not only those with a known history of trauma [4, 5]. Yet, it remains important to be skilled in asking and talking about past trauma with patients.

A number of empirically validated questionnaires related to a history of trauma exist and may be used to assess for a history of trauma exposure such as the 17-item Life Events Checklist for the DSM-5 [6]. However, no measure covers all possible experiences that could be considered traumatic to a patient (e.g., infertility, hysterectomy, pregnancy loss), some patients feel more comfortable sharing their history of trauma verbally with their healthcare professional, and follow-up of responses to any administered trauma screening instrument is necessary. Prior to the administration of any trauma screen, clinics should determine who will administer and score the screen, where the patient can privately complete the questionnaire, and who will follow-up with the patient regarding their responses and in what time frame. Additionally, a question should be included which asks patients if they are open to discussing any reported traumas with their healthcare professional.

Medical professionals have varying levels of comfort and experience managing a patient's report of trauma exposure as well as the sequelae of those experiences. It is important for healthcare professionals to be aware of their own identities (e.g., race, ethnicity, gender identity, sexuality, culture, physical/medical abilities and disabilities, neurodivergence, cognitive abilities, mental health, personality) and lived experiences (e.g., age, income, family, education, pregnancy status, body size, political beliefs, religious beliefs, trauma background), and how these impact interactions with patients (e.g., stigmatization of patient experiences). Exploration by medical professionals of their identities and lived experiences with a mental health professional can help prepare them provide high-quality trauma-informed care for their patients.

If working from a trauma-informed perspective is new to the healthcare professional, discussing past or current trauma may feel uncomfortable and/or shameful, and the presence of shame in communications with a patient can be harmful. The medical care team is encouraged to role-play with each other to build comfort in conversations surrounding trauma. Care should be taken to avoid opening the conversation with statements such as, "I am sorry to have to bring this up" as this introduces shame [7]. Instead, the medical care team should emphasize the importance of hearing and listening to patients about these important topics, with conversation starters such as, "Childhood abuse, sexual assault, and loss are common occurrences that can impact us all. I want to check in to see if you have been impacted by anything that felt traumatic to you so that you and I can work as a team to make sure you are cared for in the way that feels best for you." If trauma is disclosed, it is then imperative to listen empathically while not asking for details that are not necessary to guide care and ensuring that your statements do not minimize the patient's experience (e.g., "Thank goodness it was not worse").

Integration of Trauma Screens into Patient History Forms

All patients must complete medical histories and consent forms prior to their first visit to a new clinic. Patients may or may not respond fully to this intake paperwork, as it is unlikely they have developed a sense of trust and safety within a clinic that is unfamiliar to them. A feeling of safety and trust is important to patients who have previously experienced trauma as these experiences may have included a violation of their safety and often a betrayal of trust. However, the asking of these trauma history questions in an empathetic manner can signal to the patient that these experiences are important to and will be supported by the medical care team at the clinic. The Adverse Childhood Experiences Questionnaire for Adults (ACEs), the Life Events Checklist for the DSM-5, and/or another empirically validated measure can be included in the intake paperwork [6, 8]. Questions related to trauma exposure as a child and adult should be considered in intake paperwork and should include whether the patient has been or is currently experiencing intimate partner violence, has ever been sexually assaulted, has experienced pregnancy or infant loss, or has ever experienced medical trauma. Screening may not identify all patients with a history of trauma, and supportive psychoeducation related to trauma should be provided to encourage future disclosure of trauma. Because fertility care often spans months to years, trauma screening should be performed at multiple timepoints in the patient's care to assess for trauma which may occur during that time. Given that many people have different definitions of what counts as trauma, patients should also be asked if they have ever experienced any event that they considered to be traumatic or very upsetting.

Initial Patient Appointment

Although a patient may not feel comfortable disclosing their trauma on history forms or during verbal inquiry, if they do disclose something and indicate that they are open to talking about the experience further, it is important that it is addressed in their first patient appointment; otherwise, a patient can feel they have disclosed something important that the medical professional does not view as important. Care should be taken so that the trauma is not mentioned multiple times by different points of contact in the appointment (e.g., front desk staff, the medical assistant, the nurse, and finally, the physician). Rather, the medical team should consider ensuring that only the highest-level healthcare professional the patient will come in contact with will address the patient's trauma history.

It is also important to consider multiple factors associated with how trauma history is first introduced, taking into account SAMHSA's six key principles of TIC [2].

- The patient's sense of physical and emotional *Safety* should be attended to by considering factors such as the space in which the information is addressed to reduce the power differential. The patient should be fully clothed and, if possible, sitting at the same level as the medical professional, optimally in a warm, quiet, and private office rather than in a stark exam room where others' voices can be heard by the patient. Additionally, clinic forms should be inclusive of gender diverse identity and sexual orientation, websites and clinic spaces should include artwork and images of diverse patients, and all staff should use patient identified pronouns and names.
- *Trustworthiness and Transparency* should be addressed by using consistent welcoming eye contact, a friendly tone, emotionally validating language, accountability for clinic behaviors, and honesty and openness in communication.
- *Peer Support* options such as support groups and referrals to qualified mental health professionals should be made available for patients who disclose a history of trauma.
- *Collaboration and Mutuality* (e.g., shared respect and decision-making) are vital in this stage, as obtaining relevant information from the patient is the beginning of shared decision-making in the process of informed consent. Communication should be respectful in nature, especially when discussing differences of opinion or reasons for a medical recommendation and questions related to the healthcare professional's proposed treatment plan as compared to other treatment plans they may have learned about via other patients or social media. Collaboration also includes ongoing discussions related to informed consent for every procedure. Organizations including ACOG [9] and ASRM [10] have emphasized the importance of shared decision-making, a complete understanding of risks and benefits, the right of the patient to decline treatment, and the risks associated with declining treatment. Describe to patients all proposed procedures with each step and propose opportunities for the patient to lead care (e.g., the patient can guide speculum insertion, can insert a swab, etc.) [11]. Share with patients that (if not sedated) they can signal in an agreed-upon way (verbal or nonverbal) if they want to stop or pause a procedure and that you will check in with them during the procedure to see how they are doing. This is crucial because consent can only be given if patients also have the option of declining consent. If a patient does not consent to a recommended procedure, take care to document this with nonjudgmental language. Take care to listen to the patient for ideas on what if anything might make a procedure tolerable in the future (e.g., attending to pain related to the procedure, listening to calming music, having a support person in the room) or steps that can

be taken such as trauma-informed cognitive behavioral therapy or other mental health interventions for fear or anxiety related to medical procedures. When a patient declines to give consent, ask them when or if it is acceptable for you to ask them again about the procedure [12]. Importantly, consent should also not be viewed as a one-time signature on a piece of paper but as an ongoing process [13].

- *Empowerment, Voice, and Choice* ensure that the inherent power differential between the medical professional and the patient is attended to as the medical professional seeks to learn about what important life events have impacted the patient to better plan together for the patient's care. Additionally, healthcare professionals should recognize and validate patients' strengths, encourage patients to share their opinions, and allow patients to express their preferences with regard to treatment(s). If the patients' preferences cannot be accommodated, the healthcare professional should respectfully and transparently explain why they cannot abide by the patient's request.
- *Cultural, Historical, and Gender Issues* are an aspect of TIC that helps the medical care team be aware of and sensitive to the intersections of a patient's identities and lived experiences in providing care rather than defaulting to a "neutral" or culturally dominant perspective. In particular, awareness of the increased risk and types of traumas to which cisgender women, LGBTQ+ individuals, individuals belonging to racial/ethnic minoritized groups, disabled individuals, and those in military and other similarly structured professions are exposed can aid healthcare professionals in avoiding cultural or other biases and support patients who have experienced such traumas. Further, awareness of the stigmas of infertility and loss can help the healthcare professional re-examine their views of "needy," "angry," depressed, anxious, or otherwise "difficult" patients as patients who have instead likely felt traumatized by their reproductive experiences and potentially by other past traumas and who are in need of TIC.

Consider the following possible script at new patient visit, preferably with the patient fully clothed and in an office rather than an exam room:

> Hello, Jane it is so nice to meet you today. Before we go back to the exam room, I want to introduce myself and get to know you a little better. I am Doctor Empathy, and I have been working in this clinic for the last 4 years. Have you lived in <this city> long? I really appreciate you taking the time to fill out the paperwork before our meeting, which allowed me to review your history so we can make a plan together. [here is an opportunity to mention and ask questions about other aspects of the patient's identities and lived experiences to build understanding, trust, and rapport]. I noticed that you shared that you have experienced a sexual assault in the past and are open to discussing this experience with me.[1] I am so sorry to hear that you were assaulted. I want to make sure that you feel safe and supported while in our clinic. Are you comfortable sharing with me how long ago the assault happened? Did you receive medical care after the assault? <Do not ask for details of the assault, ensure

[1] If they say they haven't experienced an assault on their intake paperwork, you could say, I see that you indicated that you have never experienced anything traumatic such as being sexually assaulted. I know that some people don't feel comfortable saying they have been assaulted on written paperwork so I always ask patients in person (if they feel comfortable sharing with me) if they have been assaulted or if they have experienced anything else that they would consider to be traumatic in their lives.

safety, ensure your conversation makes no judgment regarding decisions of reporting or not, and check in on whether they received or would like to receive mental health or peer support. Take care not to impart shame, ensure you make eye contact, and be ready to listen empathically if they do want to share details.> Thank you for trusting me to hold that information for you. I want to make sure that you feel comfortable with the clinical care you will receive here, as I know it could include procedures such as vaginal ultrasounds and pelvic exams. I want you to know that you will always have a say in what care you receive and will play an active role in determining what is right for you. Is there anything I or we can do in the clinic to help you feel supported while you go through treatment? Are there any other experiences you have had in your life which you found to be traumatic? How are you doing emotionally coping with your diagnosis of infertility and/or experience of pregnancy loss? What questions can I answer for you?"

Key Points: Assessment of Trauma History and Application of TIC at Initial Visit

1. Include questions about trauma history in intake paperwork.
2. Grow trust through rapport-building.
3. Outline the importance of trauma-informed care.
4. Address any disclosed trauma that the patient indicates they are open to discussing, do not ask for details of the trauma, which can re-traumatize, but ensure current safety and check for the impact of trauma, listen empathically.
5. If trauma has not been disclosed on history forms, ask in person if they have experienced trauma such as sexual or physical abuse, childhood neglect, witnessing violence, experiencing medical trauma, experiencing pregnancy or infant loss, or experiencing sexual assault that they would like to share with you.
6. If trauma is disclosed, work with the patient to personalize their care, taking into account their trauma.
7. If trauma is not disclosed, ensure that care will still be taken to include the patient fully in their plan of care.
8. Include efforts to help patients feel safe, engage in transparent and collaborative communication, recognize patient strengths, and avoid stereotypes.

After the First Appointment

It is important that any treatment plan made with the patient is documented. For example, if the patient has requested that a particular type of exam not be completed or only be completed in the presence of a female healthcare professional, then this note needs to be made and highlighted in the patient's chart. The medical team should have a means of communicating a patient's preferences clearly, as a patient's trust can be significantly impacted when an agreement has been made and then this information is not noted or "gets lost" in the chart. A plan should also be made regarding how information about trauma is shared with other members of the office and medical care team. Transparency is important, so communication with the patient as to how or if they would like their trauma to be addressed by office staff and team members is important. For example, it can be important for patients that the entire staff be aware of their loss history in the REI clinic, but they may prefer to keep other traumas restricted to the medical team.

Patients may not disclose trauma in the initial contact, as again they may not feel a level of trust for this level of disclosure (or they may not feel comfortable putting it on paper). Treatment in the REI clinic can also span a length of time, wherein new trauma (e.g., pregnancy loss, negative pregnancy tests) can occur. As treatment continues, it is important to check in with patients regarding their safety and whether there are any experiences they would like to share that they feel may be impacting their well-being. By focusing on their safety and well-being, the medical team can communicate the desire to ensure the patient's needs are being met as a whole person. Continued engagement in transparent and collaborative communication with associated accountability taking, efforts to empower and support patients in the context of ongoing learning about the cultural and other issues which influence a patient's lived experience, and experience of fertility care are vital throughout the course of treatment.

Case Examples

In an effort to address the realities of practice within the REI clinic, two case examples using the same patient are presented that incorporate the trials and successes of implementing TIC.

Case Example: Regular Office Visit
Sonya arrives for her first appointment at an REI clinic and waits patiently in the waiting room. This is the first time she is going to this practice, as her long-time GYN referred her for care once it seemed that she could not assist Sonya in building her family. Sonya had difficulty finding a GYN that she could trust, and the idea of beginning again worried her. She looks around the reception area and notices that all of the chairs had armrests and look like they might be too small for her to sit comfortably in, so she stood near the receptionist's desk, filling out paperwork. Sonya and her partner have been trying for 18 months to have a baby to no avail. Her OBGYN tried six rounds of Clomid, as it was covered by insurance, which yielded one pregnancy and subsequent early miscarriage.

Sonya's name is called, and she follows the nurse to the exam room. On their way, the nurse asks Sonya to remove her shoes and step on the scale. Sonya asks if this is necessary and is told affirmatively that it is. She steps on the scale and turns her back to the register, when the nurse reads the number "225 pounds" aloud in the presence of other individuals passing in the hallway. Sonya feels shame and embarrassment as she is ushered into the exam room, told to get on the "bed" and given a paper drape and a robe with that she quickly learns doesn't fit her frame; the instructions for how to utilize these items were given with haste and she is uncertain of how to use them. She also was not told she would have a physical exam during this appointment and begins to become anxious about what procedure lies ahead of her. The doctor comes in, asks Sonya to explain why she is in the clinic today (making it clear that her doctor has not fully reviewed her medical record), briefly explains the purpose of the exam, and begins the exam. She doesn't look much at Sonya as she is frantically typing notes into her laptop. She tells Sonya that they must schedule another consultation to discuss beginning IVF with no discussion as to why IVF was recommended. Sonya is told to get dressed and return to the front desk to book her next appointment. Sonya dresses and leaves the exam room and the office, not looking back. She does not make an appointment, and she feels defeated.

This scenario contains various aspects of "business as usual" or a lack of TIC. The aesthetics of the clinic, the lack of partnering with the patient, and the focus on EMR compliance rather than constructing a physician/patient relationship are key elements where this hypothetical clinic missed the mark in creating a trauma-informed environment. It is no wonder that Sonya did not want to return. The clinic environment was not welcoming, the initial encounter with a healthcare professional was not private and communication was not transparent about the need to obtain the patient's weight or the option to not have her weight read out loud when it was clear from her physical behaviors that she did not want to know her weight, and finally, the physician's encounter with Sonya was a model of what *not* to do with a patient. Sonya's history was not reviewed with her prior to exam as recommended for TIC [14]; she was not informed ahead of time about the exam; she was not adequately consented for the exam; she felt a lack of empathy from her physician who did not review her medical record and spent most of her time typing into her laptop, and she was not queried as to any history of trauma or if there was anything that the physician could do to help her feel better during the ensuing exam.

Case Example: Invasive Procedure

Let's revisit Sonya. Upon a friend's encouragement and recommendation, Sonya tried one last time to schedule an REI consultation. She knows that she needs care and that her health needs to be important, which was not an aspect that had been modeled to her by her family. Sonya's mother had high blood pressure and high cholesterol, and her father had Type II diabetes before he died of a heart attack. In fact, Sonya's entire community seemed to avoid doctors due to a deeply held mistrust of the profession. Sonya was torn between the cultural mistrust she learned as well as the knowledge that not seeking out care could be dangerous to her.

On the day of the appointment, Sonya enters the office and in the waiting room, she sees roomy chairs, loveseats, and even a couch. She hadn't had time to complete the paperwork in advance through the portal, so she was handed an iPad at the office to complete the paperwork and was able to sit comfortably to do so. She had preferred to have an intake appointment with her new physician prior to undergoing any exams but after engaging in a supportive conversation with the scheduling team who explained that she would have a clothed conversation with her doctor prior to the exam during her appointment and could skip the exam if she didn't feel comfortable, she felt comfortable scheduling this visit. When it was time to meet with the doctor, the nurse asked her if she minded being weighed. Sonya preferred not to be weighed if it wasn't needed, and the nurse responded nonjudgmentally and guided her into the exam room, bypassing the scale altogether. She was asked to sit in a chair and remain dressed until after her initial discussion with the physician but was given a drape and an appropriately sized gown for the appointment along with thorough verbal and written instructions for how to use them.

The doctor knocked on the door a few moments later. She put her laptop to the side and sat eye-to-eye with Sonya. She explained what she had read in Sonya's medical chart and gathered a quick health history, attending to Sonya's experience with her miscarriage and checking in on any other past trauma. She then explained why the exam was indicated, with the risks and benefits of completing the exam. She asked if Sonya would like to complete the exam today. After answering a few questions that Sonya had about the exam, Sonya indicated that she consented to the exam. The physician then asked if Sonya had completed a pap smear in the past and how that experience was for her. She detailed the steps of the exam and let Sonya know that she could pause or stop the exam at any time. Sonya felt comfortable, so the healthcare professional briefly left the room while Sonya changed into her gown.

The physician knocked on the door and asked if she could come in when she returned with a chaperone and she explained that the chaperone was a trained person to ensure the exam was done properly and with consent. The doctor then asked Sonya if she was comfortable laying on the exam table and putting her feet in the footrests. As she continued the external exam, she let Sonya know what was happening and with what: for example, "This is my hand that has a glove on it, and I'm going to use it to look at your labia. Is that OK with you?" With each new aspect of the exam, the doctor patiently explained what would be occurring and asked for Sonya's consent. At one point in time, Sonya felt pressure to the point of pain. The doctor noticed her facial expression of pain and backed away, then asked if Sonya was alright and if she wanted to continue. Sonya assented, and the exam proceeded. At the end of the exam, the doctor asked Sonya if she would prefer to get dressed before they spoke about the next steps or if she wanted to do so while in her gown. Sonya chose to dress, and the nurse then escorted her to the doctor's office. The two were able to converse in the privacy of her office. Sonya was given options for fertility services that included IUI, IVF, or future options that the physician said they could speak about should they need to cross that bridge. The doctor gave Sonya some information to consider her options and told her that the office would be following up with her once she had some time to make a decision.

This visit, compared to the first example, is the polar opposite and illustrates what trauma-informed care *can* look like within an REI setting. The beginning of the encounter, as mentioned previously, begins on the phone with the scheduling team who communicated with her in a transparent manner, encouraged Sonya to be empowered to make her own choices about her care, and fostered a sense of safety and trust. A sense of safety and trust was further promoted while Sonya was in the waiting room as it was clear that the clinic recognized the importance of supporting all bodies (and eschewed weight-based stereotypes) and she was able to be comfortable as she filled out paperwork. She met with a friendly and helpful front desk staff, which continued a sense of a positive experience and started to build a sense of trust between her and the practice as a whole. The encounter with her new physician was patient-focused, and her needs were considered when the nurse bypassed taking her weight at the patient's request. During the actual exam, the physician remained attentive to her patient's body language and she frequently checked in to assess the comfort of her patient during both the external and internal portions of the exam [15]. Finally, the physician engaged in a collaborative conversation with a fully clothed Sonya after the exam to discuss future treatment options. Thus, in the above example, Sonya felt safe in the clinic which made an effort to avoid social stereotypes and stigma and began to trust clinic staff and healthcare professionals who engaged in transparent and collaborative communication which actively encouraged and empowered Sonya to have an active role in her treatment.

Trauma-Informed Delivery of Bad News

Mental health professionals are taught that "trauma is in the eye of the beholder," which is a useful way of conceptualizing a patient's unique experience of trauma, and potential activities that healthcare professionals might undertake could inadvertently contribute to a patient's experience of trauma. One of the most powerful memories that is created in patients is the moment that they receive bad news. This bad news (and whatever might follow medically regarding treatment) can become etched in the brain and can shape the events that follow in terms of the patient's experience of trauma or not [16]. Working within the fields of reproductive endocrinology as well as obstetrics and gynecology, there is no shortage of potential bad news to break, which can range from telling a patient that they ovulated early, so this cycle won't work to telling a patient that their baby's heartbeat has stopped, and so many other situations in between.

The theories around breaking bad news often come from the field of oncology and are often replicated in other specialties. Although some believe that sharing bad news is intuitive, it is actually a complex skill that, fortunately, can be taught [17]. In the field of REI, various people with differing training backgrounds might be in the position of communicating negative results, such as nurses, sonographers, and physicians, which means that more people within a clinic environment need to have a similar skill set in this area. The impact of receiving bad news can affect the relationship between the patient and practitioner, treatment choices, treatment adherence, and future healing [18].

There are multiple models of delivering bad news (e.g., [16, 18]), with each step in these models focusing on breaking bad news in a way which will be the least trauma-inducing if done correctly. For example, the SPIKES model [16] includes 6 steps each of which relates to one or more of SAMHSA's six key principles of TIC. The first step in the SPIKES model ("Setting") focuses on *safety* (e.g., creating an environment where privacy is an expectation, facilitating a support person). The second ("Perception" and third "Invitation") steps in the SPIKES model focus on *collaboration and mutuality* including understanding what the patient knows about the bad news and is on board for whatever news you have to deliver—that they want to know these results and how they best want to hear them. The fourth step ("Knowledge") focuses on *trustworthiness and transparency* through sharing the news in a way that is free of jargon, takes accountability for clinic issues, and is emotionally validating. The fifth ("Empathy/Emotion") and sixth ("Summary/Strategy") steps focus on *empowerment, voice, and choice* and allow patients the ability to share their pain; *recognize the unique cultural or other factors* which influence their experience of pain; provide an opportunity for the patient to ask any questions they may have about future treatment options; and provide an opportunity for the healthcare profession to provide referrals to *peer support* groups and mental health resources [16].

In this rapidly changing healthcare environment, systems are being put in place which enable machines to take over human tasks (e.g., breaking bad news to fertility patients). For example, patients can now receive a notification of an electronic portal message (or test results such as AMH level or pregnancy test results) and look at them prior to having spoken with their healthcare professional. On the one hand, receiving these results virtually might enable the patient to have some private time to digest the information. However, the setting a patient is in cannot be ensured (such as if the patient was at work) nor is there the ability for the patient to ask questions or feel like they are not alone. While more labor intensive, fertility patients prefer to be told bad news by a human rather than a portal message and patients may be interested in receiving referrals for mental health support during these live conversations [19, 20]. If this is not available, it might be useful to set up "office hours" where fertility patients can call or log on to speak with whoever might be available at that time to understand the portal results better.

Burnout and Compassion Fatigue

One of the difficult aspects of being a healthcare worker who works with people during some of the most difficult days of their lives is the risk of developing compassion fatigue (i.e., reduced capacity to engage in empathy due to chronic exposure to patient suffering) or burning out (i.e., a state of global exhaustion from an imbalance between organizational resources and demands which interact with individual factors) [21]. Providing TIC necessitates greater care in attending to healthcare professional self-care, as awareness and empathy of patients' trauma in itself can lead to increased exposure to vicarious trauma (i.e., negative cognitive shifts in the individual's schemas of themselves, the world, their safety, and/or others as a result of empathetic care for trauma patients) [22]. Combating these phenomena, in turn, is an integral component of trauma-informed care within a clinic or office, as these three phenomena can lead to decreased empathy, cynicism, and carelessness, which compromises patient care [23, 24]. Burnout, compassion fatigue, and vicarious traumatization are also associated with physical and mental health issues (including changes in sleeping patterns, depression, and anxiety); workplace performance and quality of care (including adverse outcomes, poor hand hygiene, and poor quality of life); and workplace attitude and behavior (including absenteeism and attrition) [21, 25].

The first step in combating compassion fatigue, burnout, and vicarious trauma is examining and implementing trauma-informed practices at the organizational level as even the most resilient practitioner will experience distress in a dysfunctional environment. This includes environments with balanced resources and demands (e.g., enough time and staff to care for patients, organizational transparency and accountability for workplace contributions to distress, collegial support, organizational tolerance of the emotional needs of its workforce, etc.) [21]. In addition to organizational interventions, individual interventions may aid in the prevention of distress. However, individual interventions in the absence of organizational change are unlikely to be effective at mitigating distress [26]. Further, it is incumbent on organizations to build resilience in their professionals as well as take a careful look at their organization and the system as well as expectations. Absent the acknowledgment of the systemic cause of distress is also likely to contribute to distress [27]. That being said, efforts to increase personal resilience can serve as a means to aid in prevention of distress within the larger organizational system of change.

There are many suggested ways in which healthcare professionals can build resilience [28] including:

1. Personal Reflection: Set long-term personal and career goals based on values, hopes, and dreams. This can be done formally in a journal or as a note on a phone.
2. Goal Setting: Make and review goals every 6 months to maintain a work–life balance in the areas of Relationships, Careers, and Hobbies/Interests. It can be useful to have an "accountability buddy"—someone with whom to share your goals and keep you on track.
3. Lifelong Learning: Engage in activities and education to improve your knowledge base and skills. This can be through CME or less formal avenues.
4. Support Network: Participate in formal organizations related to your specialty. Form relationships with colleagues for professional support. Maintain relationships with family and friends. A text/WhatsApp chain can be a lifeline.
5. Celebrate Successes and Learn from Mistakes: Professionally and personally relish even small successes and use trying times or missteps as opportunities to learn. Work to reframe mistakes as learning experiences, as humans tend to forget what they have done well.
6. Self-Care: Adequate sleep, nutrition, and joyful movement are the cornerstones of well-being. Attending to mental health via mindfulness, meditation, and personal therapy, as indicated, is also important. Again, an accountability buddy might be useful, as might a tracking app.

Conclusion

Patients seeking care in a reproductive medicine clinic are likely traumatized by their reproductive experiences and have also likely experienced other traumas in their lives. These experiences of trauma may be negatively perceived by clinic healthcare professionals and staff and/or may be re-triggered during the course of their reproductive treatment(s). Trauma-informed care is at the heart of patient-centered care and should be practiced in all fertility clinics in order to prevent patient harm and promote healing. Trauma-informed practices seek to create a safe patient environment that focuses on transparent communication with patients, empowers patients to be involved in their care and express any concerns they may have, takes accountability for any distress it causes to patients, recognizes and works to eliminate the biases and stigmas it holds about patients, and provides patients with empathetic support and access to peer support. TIC must be present during all aspects of care including scheduling, check-in, waiting areas, procedures, and consultations. Providing a trauma-informed setting not only enhances individual patient experiences but can also enhance business, as it can set practices apart. The provision of trauma-informed care also includes a focus on supporting those who treat traumatized patients and includes organizational change and accountability coupled with resilience strategies for employees.

References

1. Lawson AK, Klock SC, Pavone ME, Hirshfeld-Cytron J, Smith KN, Kazer RR. Prospective study of depression and anxiety in female fertility patients. Fertil Steril. 2014;102(5):1377–84.
2. Substance Abuse and Mental Health Services Administration. SAMHSA's concept of trauma and guidance for a trauma-informed approach. HHS publication no. (SMA) 14–4884. Rockville, MD: Substance Abuse and Mental Health Services Administration; 2014.
3. Pasch LA, Holley SR, Bleil ME, Shehab D, Katz PP, Adler NE. Addressing the needs of fertility treatment patients and their partners: are they informed of and do they receive mental health services? Fertil Steril. 2016;106(1):209–15 e2.
4. Merrick MT, Ford DC, Ports KA, Guinn AS. Prevalence of adverse childhood experiences from the 2011-2014 behavioral risk factor surveillance system in 23 states. JAMA Pediatr. 2018;172(11):1038–44.
5. Ogle CM, Rubin DC, Berntsen D, Siegler IC. The frequency and impact of exposure to potentially traumatic events over the life course. Clin Psychol Sci. 2013;1(4):426–34.
6. Weathers FW, Blake DD, Schnurr PP, Kaloupek DG, Marx BP, Keane TM. The life events checklist for DSM-5 (LEC-5)—standard. [measurement instrument]. 2013. https://www.ptsd.va.gov/.
7. Mintz LJ, Moore SE. Sexual history taking: an opportunity to reduce health disparities. J Assoc Nurs AIDS Care. 2022;33(3):241–7. https://doi.org/10.1097/JNC.0000000000000290.
8. Johnson S, Kasparian NA, Cullum AS, Flanagan T, Ponting C, Kowalewski L, Main EK. Addressing adverse childhood and adult experiences during prenatal care. Obstet Gynecol. 2023;141(6):1072–87. https://doi.org/10.1097/AOG.0000000000005199.

9. ACOG Committee. Informed consent and shared decision making in obstetrics and gynecology: ACOG Committee opinion summary, Number 819. Obstet Gynecol. 2021;137(2):392–3. https://doi.org/10.1097/aog.0000000000004248.
10. Ethics Committee of the American Society for Reproductive Medicine. Electronic address: asrm@asrm.org. Informed consent in assisted reproduction: an ethics committee opinion. Fertil Steril. 2023;119(6):948–53. https://doi.org/10.1016/j.fertnstert.2023.03.009.
11. Ireland LD, Allen RH. Pain management for gynecologic procedures in the office. Obstet Gynecol Surv. 2016;71(2):89–98. https://doi.org/10.1097/OGX.0000000000000272.
12. Farrow VA, Bosch J, Crawford JN, Snead C, Schulkin J. Screening for history of childhood abuse: beliefs, practice patterns, and barriers among obstetrician-gynecologists. Womens Health Issues. 2018;28(6):559–68. https://doi.org/10.1016/j.whi.2018.09.001.
13. Quick Safety 21. Informed consent: more than getting a signature (Updated: April 2022). Jointcommission.org. https://www.jointcommission.org/resources/news-and-multimedia/newsletters/newsletters/quick-safety/quick-safety%2D%2Dissue-21-informed%2D%2Dconsent-more-than-getting-a-signature/informed-consent-more-than-getting-a-signature/. Accessed 10 Dec 2023.
14. Demarais A, Baum N. Let your communication skills equal your clinical skills. J Med Pract Manage. 2012;28(2):116–7.
15. Tillman S. Consent in pelvic care. J Midwifery Womens Health. 2020;65(6):749–58. https://doi.org/10.1111/jmwh.13189.
16. Baile WF, Buckman R, Lenzi R, Glober G, Beale EA, Kudelka AP. SPIKES—a six-step protocol for delivering bad news: application to the patient with cancer. Oncologist. 2000;5(4):302–11. https://doi.org/10.1634/theoncologist.5-4-302.
17. Maranna S. Educating sonographers in attributes of "breaking bad news" to foster positive emotional well-being. Sonography. 2019;6(4):178–90. https://doi.org/10.1002/sono.12188.
18. Meitar D, Karnieli-Miller O. Twelve tips to manage a breaking bad news process: using S-P-w-ICE-S - a revised version of the SPIKES protocol. Med Teach. 2022;44(10):1087–91. https://doi.org/10.1080/0142159X.2021.1928618.
19. Leone D, Menichetti J, Barusi L, Chelo E, Costa M, De Lauretis L, Ferraretti AP, Livi C, Luehwink A, Tomasi G, Vegni E. Breaking bad news in assisted reproductive technology: a proposal for guidelines. Reprod Health. 2017;14(1):87. https://doi.org/10.1186/s12978-017-0350-1.
20. Mosconi L, Crescioli G, Vannacci A, Ravaldi C. Communication of diagnosis of infertility: a systematic review. Front Psychol. 2021;12:615699. https://doi.org/10.3389/fpsyg.2021.615699.
21. Forrest L, Abdurrahman M, Ritsma A. Recognizing compassion fatigue, vicarious trauma, and burnout. In: Hategan A, Saperson K, Harms S, Waters H, editors. Humanism and resilience in residency training: a guide to physician wellness. Cham: Springer; 2020.
22. Kuehn BM. Trauma-informed care may ease patient fear, clinician burnout. JAMA J Am Med Assoc. 2020;323(7):595–7. https://doi.org/10.1001/jama.2020.0052.
23. Maslach C, Jackson S. Burnout in health professions: a social psychological analysis. In: Sanders GS, Suls J, editors. Social psychology of health and illness. Hillsdale, NJ: Erlbaum; 1982.
24. Ortega MV, Hidrue MK, Lehrhoff SR, Ellis DB, Sisodia RC, Curry WT, del Carmen MG, Wasfy JH. Patterns in physician burnout in a stable-linked cohort. JAMA Netw Open. 2023;6(10):e2336745. https://doi.org/10.1001/jamanetworkopen.2023.36745.
25. Alzailai N, Barriball KL, Xyrichis A. Impact of and mitigation measures for burnout in frontline healthcare workers during disasters: a mixed-method systematic review. Worldviews Evid Based Nurs. 2023;20(2):133–41. https://doi.org/10.1111/wvn.12633.
26. Owens L, Terrell S, Low LK, Loder C, Rhizal D, Scheiman L, Seng J. Universal precautions: the case for consistently trauma-informed reproductive healthcare. Am J Obstet Gynecol. 2022;226(5):671–7. https://doi.org/10.1016/j.ajog.2021.08.012.

27. Rehder K, Adair KC, Sexton JB. The science of health care worker burnout: assessing and improving health care worker well-being. Arch Pathol Lab Med (1976). 2021;145(9):1095–109. https://doi.org/10.5858/arpa.2020-0557-RA.
28. Stubbe DE. Optimizing empathy: physician self-care as a crucial component of trauma-informed treatment. Focus. 2017;15(4):432–4. https://doi.org/10.1176/appi.focus.20170033.

Chapter 8
Strategies for Clinic Administrators and Staff

Erika L. Kelley

Successful implementation of trauma-informed care must occur across many levels, including individual, organizational/system, and community levels through an understanding of how trauma shapes behavior. Although individual healthcare professionals can implement trauma-informed care, organizational change is required to ensure that all staff are well-trained in trauma-informed principles, that trauma-informed care is effectively provided by all team members, and that staff are protected from and supported in the context of vicarious trauma (trauma symptoms developed due to the direct or indirect exposure to others' traumatic experiences). Trauma-informed organizations acknowledge the principles of trauma-informed care: trust and transparency, collaboration, choice, safety, peer support, and cultural, historical, and gender issues. Trauma-informed organizations are responsive to the needs of staff and patients/clients by embedding knowledge of the prevalence and impact of trauma within the organization's policies, procedures, and practices [1]. Trauma-informed organizations also recognize the uniqueness of their patient population(s) and acknowledge that patients may perceive diagnoses and/or medical treatment of their condition as traumatic in nature (e.g., infertility, reproductive loss). At the organization level, trauma-informed approaches focus more on relationships that are established between employees, individuals, and organizations rather than a prescribed set of interventions. There is a dearth of research regarding the implementation of trauma-informed care within reproductive endocrinology and infertility settings specifically. However, research and theory from the broader

E. L. Kelley (✉)
Division of Behavioral Medicine, Department of OB/GYN, University Hospitals Cleveland Medical Center, Cleveland, OH, USA

Departments of Reproductive Biology and Urology, School of Medicine, Case Western Reserve University, Cleveland, OH, USA

MacDonald Women's Hospital, Cleveland, OH, USA
e-mail: Erika.Kelley@UHhospitals.org

A. Lawson, A. Swanson (eds.), *Trauma-Informed Reproductive Healthcare*,
https://doi.org/10.1007/978-3-031-67474-7_8

literature can be utilized to provide guidance to administrators and staff in these settings. Overall, the principles of trauma-informed care can be used to guide organization- and staff-level decisions, behaviors, policies, procedures, and practices. The application of strategies described herein will vary depending on the size, setting, and makeup of the specific clinical practice or organization.

The content discussed in this chapter may be relevant to both administrators and staff. Administrators are positioned to attend to the needs of both staff and patients/clients through implementation of the trauma-informed care principles. They can serve as leaders in the effort toward successful trauma-informed care across the organization. Staff at all levels can engage in efforts to promote trauma-informed care across the organization. Administrators and staff who work in clinical settings set within larger organizations may be in a position of advocating to leaders of the organization for support in incorporating trauma-informed care across the system.

Organization/Clinic-Level Policies and Procedures

Administrators can ensure that trauma-informed care principles are embedded within the vision, mission, culture, policies, and procedures of the clinic or organization in a variety of ways. These documents and procedures should be evaluated and updated on a regular basis to incorporate new information from the field of trauma-informed care, to be responsive to changing needs of the staff and community served, and to ensure that trauma-informed care elements are considered within any practice-level changes. Successful application of these efforts necessitates an understanding of how trauma impacts a specific population that the practice serves. As described in other sections of this book, there are a variety of ways in which patients seeking reproductive endocrinology and infertility (REI) care may experience trauma. An administrative- and organization-level understanding of the community within which an organization or practice is embedded is important. This is consistent with the trauma-informed care principle of “cultural, historical, and gender issues,” such that an organization works to move beyond cultural biases, is culturally responsive, and recognizes the impact of historical trauma [1]. To this end, it may be beneficial for patients, staff, and community members to sit on advisory boards to help inform system-level policies and procedures.

The organization’s practice and procedural guidelines should provide guidance surrounding trauma-informed care and provide clear expectations, communication, and definitions of trauma-informed care for all staff [2]. For example, procedures regarding screening for trauma history in patients/clients should be clear and used consistently across healthcare professionals. As another example, policies that prohibit having a significant other in an exam and/or operating room may be made flexible for individuals with a trauma history. Allowing a partner or other support person to be present and provide additional support to the client/patient during embryo transfer, rather than having them wait in the waiting or recovery room, may reduce psychological distress. In psychological and/or ethical guidelines used in patient/client care (e.g., for treatments involving egg or sperm donors, or gestational carriers), guidelines related to patients with trauma histories should be considered. Patients/clients may worry that their history of exposure to interpersonal violence or experience of associated mental health symptoms (e.g., post-traumatic stress disorder) will affect their candidacy for ART or involvement as a donor or GC. Clarity regarding if/when such psychosocial and medical history will be assessed and what impact it may or may not have on care (e.g., impact of untreated mental illness) should be made clear. In addition, trauma-informed care elements can be beneficial to consider when screening for such histories or providing feedback about the implications of such histories. When developing informed consent for treatment procedures, the clinic may consider how to explain to patients if and/or why trauma history and mental health information is being asked and how it may (or may not) affect treatment (e.g., clarification of if/how disclosure of trauma history affects psychological candidacy or treatment plan). Considering the importance of trust and privacy in trauma-informed care, asking sensitive information with no explanation as to why it is solicited may be particularly triggering for patients who have a history of trauma. Thus, clear informed consent processes should be consistently incorporated throughout the clinic [3].

Local safety strategies and policies, specific to the organization and setting, should be constructed, such as having adequate lighting for parking lots, garages, and hallways and/or trauma-informed security officers present on site [4]. These should be informed by all stakeholders (e.g., healthcare professionals, staff, leadership, and clients) to address the safety needs specific to that setting. Furthermore, systems (e.g., patient advocacy offices, ombudsmen) should be in place to allow for safe reporting of, and responses to, incidents where trauma-informed care was not appropriately implemented. Development and maintenance of a trauma-informed organization must be considered from a financial perspective and built into budgetary decisions [1]. Moreover, providing staff with increased access to the organization's strategic information, policies, and procedures can promote transparency and lower levels of vicarious traumatization [5, 6].

Building a Trauma-Informed Team

Hiring Elements of trauma-informed care should be considered during the employee recruitment and hiring process [1]. Administrators should ensure that incoming staff have training in trauma-informed care and/or are open to receiving training in this area and are committed to the principles of trauma-informed care [7]. Interviews of job candidates can include questions on this topic. Employee roles and responsibilities should be clearly outlined as a form of transparency [8]. Staff should be educated about the specific populations with whom they will work and about possible risks associated with working with survivors of trauma, such as vicarious trauma [4]. Relatedly, exit interviews can be valuable opportunities to receive feedback about organizational efforts to engage in trauma-informed care and reduce vicarious traumatization and burnout [7].

Administrators may consider hiring mental/behavioral health care professionals with appropriate expertise and training in REI. Given the complex psychosocial issues experienced by fertility patients/clients, there is a need for trained fertility counselors who can assist both patients/clients and staff. Mental/behavioral health care professionals with expertise in fertility counseling can provide needed psychotherapeutic interventions and support for individuals and couples facing fertility challenges, those using ART for fertility preservation or family building, and/or those using third-party reproduction services. Psychological assessment is also recommended for determination of candidacy for those seeking involvement in third-party reproduction [9]. Many REI settings work with mental health professionals as part of the interdisciplinary approach [9]; thus, recruiting mental health professionals who are trained both in the area of REI and trauma-informed care may be particularly helpful. When possible, this interdisciplinary approach should be considered in payment systems used, through integrating physical and behavioral health services financing to reduce the financial burden of mental health care and other barriers to care for patients/clients [2]. Alternatively, having a trusted referral network, facilitating warm hand-offs to those resources/referrals, and having an established relationship with community organizations to support clients can promote trauma-informed care [1].

Staff Schedules When developing healthcare professionals' and staff schedules, strategies for providing adequate, regular breaks should be identified to promote well-being [10, 11]. Reproductive nurses in particular may have significant exposure to patient trauma as they are often on the front line of speaking with traumatized patients about failed treatments and reproductive losses. Particular attention should be paid to the well-being of fertility clinic staff exposed to the greatest amount of patient reproductive and other trauma(s). Patient/client caseloads can be balanced with regard to working with trauma survivors (and within populations where the prevalent diagnoses and treatment may be considered traumatic, such as in reproductive medicine) when possible [6, 10]. Variation of job duties can also lessen burnout [12]. Administrators may also monitor staff and employee time off and encourage employees who accrue too much time to take time off [4]. The structure of clinic scheduling may also need to take into account allowing time for longer visits and/or more follow-up visits for individuals with a trauma history, which might require scheduling and/or billing changes. An additional consideration is that socioeconomic factors may impact a patients'/clients' ability to attend or afford these additional or longer visits.

Physical Environment

All aspects of the physical environment a patient/client or staff member may encounter should be considered from a trauma-informed care lens, when possible. An environment that promotes safety, privacy, trust, empowerment, collaboration, and choice is ideal [1, 13]. Both psychological and physical safety should be prioritized. When constructing a clinical or work space, administrators and staff may incorporate elements of trauma-informed design, which focuses on the physical environment from a trauma-informed care perspective [14, 15].

Creating a warm, neat, efficient, calming, and welcoming space is important [16]. Staff should consider minimizing excess clutter (e.g., piles of paperwork or boxes) that may be distracting or overstimulating to both staff and clients alike. Art can be placed in client areas as a source of visual comfort, while making sure it is not triggering to the specific patient population (e.g., pictures of babies may generate feelings of sadness or anger in individuals diagnosed with infertility, failure to include art which represents the identities of a broad reproductive patient population may feel exclusionary and lead patients to worry about their safety in the clinic). Allowing art in staff spaces can also promote overall self-care and well-being [4]. Excess "noise" should be minimized (e.g., a buzzing light, loud air conditioner, or multiple televisions on in a waiting room), as this can increase anxiety [16]. Organization of waiting rooms should also take into account the specific patient population. For example, having separate waiting rooms for pregnant patients and those in treatment for infertility can be helpful.

Selecting furniture and decorations that are calming can contribute to a trauma-informed care space [13]. For example, selecting cool color schemes (e.g., blues, greens) and avoiding "harsh" (e.g., reds, oranges) or overly-stark or "sterile" white designs can be calming. Light-colored rooms create a sense of openness, which may appear safer. Placing furniture which accomodates all body sizes in such a way where the patient can see and easily access the exit, and minimizing crowding when arranging seating may be beneficial. Allowing for natural lighting and air should be balanced with the need for privacy (e.g., considering whether or not to open windows or blinds if clinical conversations might be overheard or seen from outside). The interrelationship between physical and psychological safety can be seen in many strategies described herein. For example, in examination rooms, placing examination tables facing away from the door may allow patients/clients to feel less exposed and having an easily accessed exit may allow them to feel less trapped.

In spaces where clinical care is provided, strategies to ensure that confidentiality is maintained is important. Staff should make sure not to discuss patient information in any spaces that are not secure and confidential. When patients are waiting in an exam or office room and overhear the doctor–patient conversation in the next room, this creates an unsafe space when they suspect their own appointment will be overheard. Thus, adequate sound-proofing reduces the likelihood that someone could overhear clinical conversations. Strategies such as white-noise machines and spacing of office rooms that reduce (and ideally eliminate) potential to be overheard should be considered. This is also important to consider in procedure suites where patients may overhear information about another patient's pre- or post-procedural care (e.g., how many oocytes were retrieved for another patient, treatment complications, difficulty arousing from anesthesia, etc.). In check-in areas, strategies to maintain privacy should be implemented. Examples include not leaving patient sign-in sheets visible to others and providing enough space so check-in conversations are not overheard. Privacy screens for computer monitors can minimize the likelihood that patient information on the screen is viewed by others. In addition, information about patient rights and responsibilities should be clearly posted in the clinic to promote transparency. Content (e.g., posters, brochures) about trauma and coping mechanisms for use within the reproductive health care setting can be posted to build awareness and allow clients to know it is a safe space [13].

Telemedicine Procedures

Trauma-informed care should be provided regardless of the location in which such treatment occurs thus, an organization's standard operating procedures for provision of telemedicine should also incorporate trauma-informed care elements [17]. If providing telemedicine services, clinics should provide sufficient information ahead of time to the patient about how privacy, security, and confidentiality is ensured when using such technologies. For example, patients with a trauma history may be particularly likely to worry that a session is being recorded or overheard by others. As additional examples of how to incorporate trauma-informed care in telemedicine procedures, policies can include requirements for the healthcare professional or staff member's camera to be turned on when possible, and allowing the patient to see that the healthcare professional or staff member is in a secure, private space such that their conversation is not overheard. Healthcare professionals should use headphones to demonstrate confidentiality and psychological safety. Providing a consent or informational sheet prior to the appointment that clearly describes whether or when sessions are recorded, and who is in the virtual "room" promotes safety and trust.

Training for Staff

Trauma-informed care training should be provided to all members of the organization appropriate to that person's role, and should be facilitated on a regular, recurring basis (at least annually) [1, 4, 18, 19]. Education and training on trauma and trauma-informed care should be available for anyone who may encounter patients within the organization. For example, individuals beyond staff who provide direct patient care such as patient access representatives, front desk personnel, and scribes should be included. Security personnel, parking valets or attendants, and housekeeping staff may benefit from knowledge of trauma-informed care not only regarding interactions with clients, but also in considering the physical environment of the organization (e.g., ensuring entrances, hallways, and garages are well-lit). Patient advocacy staff members, ombudsmen, and individuals in similar positions should be provided trauma-informed care training. Even if in-depth training is not possible or available, staff members can be provided basic strategies for offering validation of patient experiences and establishment of safety, trust, and privacy. Furthermore, organizations that work with health care trainees (e.g., fellows and residents) and students should consider providing formal training in trauma-informed care to these individuals, given some research indicating insufficient trauma-informed care training in residency programs [20, 21].

In addition, individuals who provide services to populations experiencing trauma are at risk of vicarious traumatization [22, 23]. Vicarious traumatization leads to negative and/or distressing changes in cognitive, emotional, and behavioral experiences as a result of directly caring for individuals with a trauma history (see later section). Briefly, administrators should provide opportunities for sufficient education about vicarious trauma and support to all staff members. Education about vicarious trauma and burnout and opportunities for support should be provided in all new staff orientation, and then provided at regular intervals with updated information (at least annually). Organizations can increase awareness (and if budget allows, make available) resources such as books, webinars, and trainings on both trauma-informed care and vicarious trauma-informed care.

As noted previously, successful and lasting trauma-informed care implementation can take years and requires ongoing efforts for sustainability. It is not a one-size-fits-all intervention or simple "checklist" but rather a continual process across time [1] and administrators should plan accordingly. The specific training modality will depend on the current culture of the organization and status of trauma-informed care implementation at the institution. When training staff and health care professionals, administrators must consider the financial impact as time spent on training does not produce immediate revenue. However, this short-term loss of revenue will likely be offset by the longer-term improvement in care, reductions in health care costs (e.g., reduction of ER visits, reduced number of visits due to multi-morbidity), and reduced patient drop-out when trauma-informed care is appropriately provided as the provision of patient-centered care has been shown to increase patient satisfaction in fertility patients [24]. In addition to benefits for patients/clients, trauma-informed care and vicarious trauma-informed care approaches within an organization can lead to increased staff retention, higher quality of service delivery, and improved employee well-being [25]. Some research indicates that common barriers to trauma-informed care training include lack of available time and lack of access to trained facilitators [21]. Thus, administrators may need to consider hiring trainers with expertise in trauma-informed care who are external to the organization or sending employees to external trainings, which should be considered in budget and schedule planning. Implementation coaching following training supports successful implementation of the training and is offered by some organizations that provide training and support for organization-level implementation of trauma-informed care. In addition, if implementing trauma-informed care training, mechanisms should be in place to evaluate the impact of this training.

There are multiple models of trauma-informed training and many organizations that provide trauma-informed resources and training to support lasting trauma-informed care practices and culture within health care settings. Examples include: resources from the Traumatic Stress Institute (https://www.traumaticstressinstitute.org), SAMHSA's National Center for Trauma-Informed Care (https://www.traumainformedcare.chcs.org/resource/samhsas-national-center-for-trauma-informed-care/) and models described within Grossman et al.'s discussion of example approaches [26]. The Center for Health Care Strategies is a policy and implementation partner that focuses on improving outcomes for people enrolled in Medicaid and provides trauma-informed care implementation resources (https://www.traumainformedcare.chcs.org/). Furthermore, the Office of Victims of Crime has a toolkit of resources specifically for supporting vicarious trauma-informed organizations (https://ovc.ojp.gov/program/vtt/tools-for-victim-services#u7eb0g). This list is by no means exhaustive, and with the increasing recognition of the importance of trauma-informed care will likely continue to grow.

Vicarious Trauma

Individuals who work directly or indirectly with trauma survivors may experience a multitude of psychological reactions as a result of exposure to descriptions of patients' trauma histories and sometimes in vivo witnessing of a patient's trauma (e.g., presence during an ultrasound confirming a pregnancy loss). Some research demonstrates ways in which working with trauma survivors can be rewarding. For example, working with trauma survivors can lead to positive changes in perspectives, goals, and priorities and satisfaction when helping someone recover from a trauma [27, 28]. Unfortunately, employees are also at risk for the development of vicarious traumatization, compassion fatigue or secondary traumatic stress, and burnout.

Vicarious traumatization results from working directly with individuals who experienced trauma and is a transformation of cognitive, behavioral, and emotional experiences within an employee. This can particularly lead to changes in beliefs about safety, power, trust, control, and esteem [19, 22, 23, 29–31]. A similar concept, compassion fatigue (at times interchangeably used with secondary traumatic stress), is an acute emotional crisis that can occur through direct or indirect exposure to work with trauma survivors and has been explored among health care professionals across a variety of settings [32, 33]. Symptoms appear similar to the symptoms of post-traumatic stress disorder (PTSD) and include re-experiencing symptoms (e.g., intrusive thoughts about a patient's trauma history), alterations in mood (e.g., excessive anger or fear), hyperarousal symptoms (e.g., sleep disruption), and avoidance and numbing (e.g., avoiding internal or external reminders of patient's trauma histories) [32–35]. Burnout can occur outside of the context of working with trauma survivors, and can occur in response to prolonged strain from professional (e.g., ongoing work with trauma populations; heavy patient load) and/or personal (e.g., caring for a loved one who is ill) stress. Burnout is often a progressive process when stress results in emotional exhaustion, decreased feelings of mastery or accomplishment, and an inability to separate from or depersonalize client experiences [36]. Vicarious trauma and compassion fatigue may contribute to burnout [18].

Providing Support for Staff Health and Wellness

Vicarious Trauma Education and Assessment Vicarious trauma and increased stress levels among employees can negatively impact work performance, and ultimately health and well-being. In terms of work performance, vicarious trauma and stress can negatively affect staff decision-making abilities and their interactions with clients and coworkers [37, 38]. Vicarious trauma, stress, and burnout among employees can also lead to employee turnover, reduced productivity, and negative effects on team cohesion and collaboration [38]. This provides further support for the longer-term benefit of preventing and addressing vicarious trauma even if those efforts result in short-term loss of productivity. Administrators should provide education to staff members about these concepts and encourage efforts to prevent and/or mitigate them. Without an understanding of what these concepts are, healthcare professionals and staff may subsequently experience thoughts of self-blame, shame, or guilt (e.g., "what's wrong with me that I am feeling this way"). Making explanations of these concepts available to staff can provide a sense of validation and increased awareness. Education surrounding vicarious trauma and burnout can be embedded within annual training regarding trauma-informed care.

Administrators should provide an infrastructure that supports open communication about preventing and addressing vicarious trauma, and support a work environment that promotes safety, trust, choice, empowerment, and collaboration. This can be done a variety of ways. For example, via regular team meetings, private supervision meetings with individual staff members, or a point person trained in trauma-informed care who can solicit feedback on this topic. Performance or competency evaluations can include questions related to burnout and vicarious traumatization (with the option to leave these items blank to protect staff concerns about personal job security should they disclose burnout or traumatization) and be discussed privately and/or voluntarily. A mechanism for debriefing following difficult work interactions (e.g., negative patient outcomes) should be made available routinely to staff [18]. If implementing interventions or strategies to prevent or reduce vicarious trauma and burnout, efforts should be made to evaluate these efforts at least annually and for employees to provide feedback about them [12]. As an example, some research demonstrates the benefit of the Stress Management and Resiliency Training (SMART) program, which aims to reduce responses to stress and teaches resiliency enhancement among health care professionals [39, 40]. Other models exist and are being developed and evaluated for addressing these issues in various health care settings [e.g., [41]].

Administrators may also provide voluntary opportunities for staff to complete self-assessment measures to screen for elevated levels of vicarious trauma, compassion fatigue, and/or burnout. Example measures include the Professional Quality of Life Scale (ProQOL) [42, 43] that assesses positive and negative impacts of working with trauma populations and the Maslach Burnout Inventory [44] that assesses emotional exhaustion, depersonalization, and personal accomplishment. These measures should be completed privately by staff and employees who wish to complete them. Transparency as to how the organization may respond to staff reports of burnout, stress, and/or vicarious trauma should be provided to staff prior to survey completion. Retaliatory or punitive organizational responses are never appropriate and likely create a chilling effect, which reduces staff comfort in discussing their well-being with their employer. Organizations can provide support by making these measures known and available, and offering voluntary and confidential opportunities for discussion of employees' results on these scales, provided that the work environment is perceived as a safe space [6, 18].

Team Support Having a safe, supportive team environment to process and discuss vicarious trauma and having structured protocols for case review and debriefing is crucial [4]. It is equally crucial to recognize and respect that not all attendees of case reviews and debriefings may feel comfortable sharing their feelings and reactions. Pressuring staff to share their inner experiences should be avoided. When indicated, training and supervision should provide a supportive and safe space to discuss vicarious traumatization [6, 12]. Creating opportunities for formal and informal social gatherings among staff can help reduce stress, burnout, and vicarious trauma [4]. Administrators may also consider partnering with organizations that focus on work with trauma survivors for additional support and information sharing [2, 22].

Health and Wellness Administrators should provide resources and opportunities to address vicarious trauma and reduce the potential impact of burnout among staff. The types of opportunities provided may vary depending on the size of the organization and the resources available. In addition, these may need to be planned in advance with consideration of budget and clinic schedules (e.g., ensuring sufficient clinical coverage if staff are engaging in wellness activities during office hours). Administrators should encourage staff to practice self-care during personal and work time [4, 18]. When possible, organizations should provide access to health and wellness activities, such as yoga, mindfulness, and fitness programs [45]. As another example, organizations may implement incentive programs to reward employee engagement in wellness activities, and may provide monthly 'mental health days' off to staff. Coverage of mental health services should be provided to employees when possible [4]. It should be noted, that efforts to improve health and wellness in the absence of balanced work-related resources and demands is likely insufficient to prevent burnout.

In short, administrators and staff have a responsibility to patients to understand the prevalence and impact of trauma within the community they serve. There are many ways in which clinic administrators and staff can be leaders, advocates, and facilitators of trauma-informed care across an organization.

DisclaimerThe views expressed in this chapter are those of the author and do not necessarily reflect the position or policy of the American Society for Reproductive Medicine, or the US government.

References

1. Administration SAaMHS. SAMHSA's concept of trauma and guidance for a trauma-informed approach. Rockville, MD: Substance Abuse and Mental Health Services Administration; 2014.
2. Menschner C, Maul A. Issue brief: key ingredients for successful trauma-informed care implementation. Hamilton: Center for Health Care Strategies; 2016.
3. Rudolph K. Ethical considerations in trauma-informed care. Psychiatr Clin North Am. 2021;44(4):521–35.
4. Bell H, Kulkarni S, Dalton L. Organizational prevention of vicarious trauma. Fam Soc. 2003;84(4):463–70.
5. Choi G-Y. Organizational impacts on the secondary traumatic stress of social workers assisting family violence or sexual assault survivors. Adm Soc Work. 2011;35(3):225–42.
6. Sutton L, Rowe S, Hammerton G, Billings J. The contribution of organisational factors to vicarious trauma in mental health professionals: a systematic review and narrative synthesis. Eur J Psychotraumatol. 2022;13(1):2022278.
7. Team TVP, Practice tNUIoUHRa. Human resource guidelines for a vicarious trauma-informed organization. 2016.
8. Adams K, Shakespeare-Finch J, Armstrong D. An interpretive phenomenological analysis of stress and well-being in emergency medical dispatchers. J Loss Trauma Int Perspect Stress Coping. 2015;20(5):430–48.
9. Medicine PCatMHPGotASfR. Guidance on qualifications for fertility counselors: a committee opinion. Fertil Steril. 2021;115:1411–5.
10. Baird S, Jenkins SR. Vicarious traumatization, secondary traumatic stress, and burnout in sexual assault and domestic violence agency staff. Violence Vict. 2003;18(1):71–86.
11. Donisch K, Bray C, Gewirtz A. Child welfare, juvenile justice, mental health, and education providers' conceptualizations of trauma-informed practice. Child Maltreat. 2016;21(2):125–34.
12. White D. The hidden costs of caring: what managers need to know. Health Care Manag (Frederick). 2006;25(4):341–7.
13. Council NHCftH. Creating a culture of safety: a guide for health centers. 2017.
14. Ajeen R, Ajeen D, Wisdom JP, Greene JA, Lepage T, Sjoelin C, et al. The impact of trauma-informed design on psychological Well-being in homeless shelters. Psychol Serv. 2022;20:680.
15. Wilson C, Pence D, Conradi L. Trauma-informed care. Encyclopedia of social work. NASW Press and Oxford University Press; 2013. p. 1–22.
16. Care NIfMR. Checklist for creating a trauma-informed environment in medical respite. National Health Care for the Homeless Council; 2023.
17. Gerber MR, Elisseou S, Sager ZS, Keith JA. Trauma-informed telehealth in the COVID-19 era and beyond. Fed Pract. 2020;37(7):302–8.
18. Sansbury BS, Graves K, Scott W. Managing traumatic stress responses among clinicians: individual and organizational tools for self-care. Trauma. 2015;17(2):114–22.

19. Burns CJ, Borah L, Terrell SM, James LN, Erkkinen E, Owens L. Trauma-informed Care curricula for the health professions: a scoping review of best practices for design, implementation, and evaluation. Acad Med. 2023;98(3):401–9.
20. DeAndrade S, Pelletier A, Grossman S, Lewis-O'Connor A, Royce C, Dutton C, et al. Trauma-informed care training in Ob/gyn residency [26g]. Obstet Gynecol. 2020;135:77S.
21. Dichter ME, Teitelman A, Klusaritz H, Maurer DM, Cronholm PF, Doubeni CA. Trauma-informed Care training in family Medicine residency programs results from a CERA survey. Fam Med. 2018;50(8):617–22.
22. McCann IL, Pearlman LA. Vicarious traumatization: a framework for understanding the psychological effects of working with victims. J Trauma Stress. 1990;3:131–49.
23. Pearlman L, Saakvitne K. Treating therapists with vicarious traumatization and secondary traumatic stress disorders. In: Figley C, editor. Compassion fatigue: coping with secondary traumatic stress disorder in those who treat the traumatized. Florence, KY: Brunner/Mazel; 1995. p. 150–77.
24. Shandley LM, Hipp HS, Anderson-Bialis J, Anderson-Bialis D, Boulet SL, McKenzie LJ, et al. Patient-centered care: factors associated with reporting a positive experience at United States fertility clinics. Fertil Steril. 2020;113(4):797–810.
25. Team TVP, College WJ. Making the business case for a vicarious trauma-informed organization. 2016.
26. Grossman S, Cooper Z, Buxton H, Hendrickson S, Lewis-O'Connor A, Stevens J, et al. Trauma-informed care: recognizing and resisting re-traumatization in health care. Trauma Surg Acute Care Open. 2021;6(1):e000815.
27. Råbu M, Moltu C, Binder PE, McLeod J. How does practicing psychotherapy affect the personal life of the therapist? A qualitative inquiry of senior therapists' experiences. Psychother Res. 2016;26(6):737–49.
28. Killian K, Hernandez-Wolfe P, Engstrom D, Gangsei D. Development of the vicarious resilience scale (VRS): a measure of positive effects of working with trauma survivors. Psychol Trauma. 2017;9(1):23–31.
29. Sinclair HA, Hamill C. Does vicarious traumatisation affect oncology nurses? A literature review. Eur J Oncol Nurs. 2007;11(4):348–56.
30. Sabin-Farrell R, Turpin G. Vicarious traumatization: implications for the mental health of health workers? Clin Psychol Rev. 2003;23(3):449–80.
31. Devilly GJ, Wright R, Varker T. Vicarious trauma, secondary traumatic stress or simply burnout? Effect of trauma therapy on mental health professionals. Aust N Z J Psychiatry. 2009;43(4):373–85.
32. Bride BE. Prevalence of secondary traumatic stress among social workers. Soc Work. 2007;52(1):63–70.
33. Figley C. Treating compassion fatigue. New York, NY: Brunner-Routledge; 2002.
34. Smith AJ, Kleijn WC, Trijsburg RW, Hutschemaekers GJ. How therapists cope with clients' traumatic experiences. Torture. 2007;17(3):203–15.
35. Ravaldi C, Mosconi L, Mannetti L, Checconi M, Bonaiuti R, Ricca V, et al. Post-traumatic stress symptoms and burnout in healthcare professionals working in neonatal intensive care units: results from the STRONG study. Front Psych. 2023;14:1050236.
36. Maslach C. Burnout: the cost of caring. Los Altos, CA: Malor Books; 2015.
37. Stebnicki MA. Psychosocial impact of empathy fatigue on professional helpers. In: Stebnicki M, Marini I, editors. Psychological and social impact of illness and disability. 6th ed. New York, NY: Springer; 2012. p. 423–34.
38. Knight C. Indirect trauma: implications for self-care, supervision, the organization, and the academic institution. Clin Superv. 2013;32(2):224–43.
39. Park ER, Traeger L, Vranceanu AM, Scult M, Lerner JA, Benson H, et al. The development of a patient-centered program based on the relaxation response: the relaxation response resiliency program (3RP). Psychosomatics. 2013;54(2):165–74.

40. Dossett ML, Needles EW, Nittoli CE, Mehta DH. Stress management and resiliency training for healthcare professionals: a mixed-methods, quality-improvement, cohort study. J Occup Environ Med. 2021;63(1):64–8.
41. Allen R, Watt F, Jansen B, Coghlan E, Nathan EA. Minimising compassion fatigue in obstetrics/gynaecology doctors: exploring an intervention for an occupational hazard. Australas Psychiatry. 2017;25(4):403–6.
42. Stamm B. Measuring compassion satisfaction as well as fatigue: developmental history of the compassion fatigue and satisfaction test. In: Figley C, editor. Treating compassion fatigue. New York, NY: Brunner/Mazel; 2002. p. 107–19.
43. Stamm BH. The concise ProQOL manual. 2nd ed. Pocatello, ID: ProQOL.org; 2010.
44. Maslach C. The Maslach burnout inventory. 3rd ed. Palo Alto, CA: Consulting Psychologists Press; 1996.
45. Thieleman K, Cacciatore J. Witness to suffering: mindfulness and compassion fatigue among traumatic bereavement volunteers and professionals. Soc Work. 2014;59(1):34–41.

Chapter 9
The Role of the Mental Health Professional

Teni Davoudian

Overview of Contributions

The contributions of reproductive mental health professionals (MHPs) to the field of reproductive medicine have evolved and expanded over the past four decades [1]. Qualified MHPs now provide clinical services to patients prior to, during, and following fertility and other treatments for reproductive concerns. The loss of control over one's reproductive options and status is often accompanied by significant psychological distress. In fact, studies have found that infertility can be as stressful as having cancer and congestive heart failure [2, 3]. The American Society for Reproductive Medicine (ASRM) recognizes the complex emotional landscape of reproductive challenges and recommends that clinics utilizing assisted reproductive technologies include an embedded mental health professional or establish a consultancy relationship with an external MHP [4].

Many reproductive medicine patients are faced with navigating the substantial emotional burdens of the diagnosis and treatment of reproductive concerns/conditions (e.g., infertility, pregnancy loss) while also managing pre-existing or newly developed mental health condition(s). Common psychological comorbidities to infertility include major depressive disorder, generalized anxiety disorder, and post-traumatic stress disorder (PTSD; [5, 6]). Infertility and assisted reproductive technologies are known to increase the risk of PTSD [7]. It should also be noted that not all reproductive experiences which fertility patients consider to be traumatic (e.g., being diagnosed with infertility, being unable to have a child) qualify for a diagnosis of PTSD but these experiences may still feel traumatizing and lead to significant psychological distress.

T. Davoudian (✉)
Oregon Health and Science University, Portland, OR, USA
e-mail: davoudia@ohsu.edu; teni.davoudian@bcm.edu

A. Lawson, A. Swanson (eds.), *Trauma-Informed Reproductive Healthcare*,
https://doi.org/10.1007/978-3-031-67474-7_9

Given the high prevalence of distress, trauma and PTSD among reproductive medicine patients [8], it is imperative for MHPs in the field of reproductive medicine to not only meet the qualifications of fertility counselors [9], but also possess extensive knowledge about PTSD and trauma, including reproductive traumas. MPHs with appropriate training and supervision in both reproductive medicine and PTSD should strive to provide evidence-based treatments for trauma that are sensitive to the needs of this specific patient population.

In addition to trauma-informed patient care, qualified MHPs can help promote trauma-informed approaches to patient care by serving as educators and/or consultants to reproductive medicine clinics. This role can entail facilitating workshops for reproductive endocrinology trainees, medical teams, and staff regarding the diagnosis of PTSD, consequences of trauma exposure, and provision of trauma-informed patient care. MHPs can also help establish psychological symptom screening protocols, provide trauma-informed referrals/sources, and assess outcomes of trauma-informed approaches within fertility clinics.

Universal Screening

Currently, there are no standardized policies regarding the universal screening of trauma in adult healthcare settings [10]. Various barriers, such as insufficient resources, limited time with patients, and lack of personnel may impede trauma inquiries. However, screening all patients for posttraumatic stress disorder and other symptoms of psychological distress is considered to be best practice and the first step to providing quality patient care [11]. Sensitive inquiry into patients' trauma and emotional history is also critical when it comes to referring patients to appropriate resources.

MHPs with appropriate training in trauma-informed care can serve as consultants to clinics interested in implementing or improving their trauma and psychological screening procedures. Qualified MHPs can help ensure that the principles of trauma-informed care, such as safety, choice, and transparency, are considered and applied when deciphering the logistics of the screening process. For example, psychoeducation about trauma and screening for traumas should occur in a private area and patients should be fully dressed while screened. All patients should also be given the choice and give informed consent to participate in screening procedures. Furthermore, screening should be inclusive of all current and past psychological distress/experiences as it is well known that both past and more recent traumatic experiences can affect current emotional well-being [12]. Furthermore, focusing solely on current PTSD symptomatology may inappropriately send the message that only current PTSD symptoms are worthy of discussion/concern. This may therefore inadvertently stigmatize the experience of trauma and PTSD, limit healthcare professionals' greater understanding of the patient's emotional well-being and personal psychological risks associated with infertility and/or its treatment, and hinder the provision of care or referrals needed to best support patients.

MHPs can also ensure that the measures utilized by reproductive medicine clinics to screen for psychological distress (including PTSD) have been standardized and tested for their psychometric soundness. When possible, questionnaires should be provided to patients in their preferred language (e.g., the Posttraumatic Checklist-5 is currently available in 12 languages) and psychoeducation about the importance of screenings should be provided [13]. MHPs can also review and discuss the potential strengths/limitations of the assessment tools selected by the clinic and assist in the development of follow-up procedures for patients who report experiences of trauma and/or psychological distress. It should be noted that following disclosure of trauma and/or psychological distress, some patients may experience emotional dysregulation while others may find that disclosure within a validating and emotionally safe environment has therapeutic value. MHPs should therefore model to staff and healthcare professionals various empathic, validating responses (both verbal and non-verbal) to the disclosure of trauma and/or psychological distress. MHPs should also share with healthcare professionals strategies for coping with the experience of vicarious trauma (i.e., psychological distress experienced as a result of witnessing or hearing about someone else's experience of trauma), which is discussed further in a different section of this chapter.

PTSD, Trauma, and Psychological Distress in the Context of Reproductive Healthcare

Many healthcare professionals hesitate to inquire about or respond to patients' trauma histories or experiences of psychological distress due to limited trauma-specific knowledge and insufficient training on how to therapeutically manage such interactions [14]. MHPs with appropriate proficiency in the presentation and treatment of psychological distress including PTSD can offer educational sessions to clinical and non-clinical staff at reproductive medicine clinics. In fact, MHPs may be particularly skilled at creating an environment of safety and acceptance during staff educational sessions given their training and consistent practice in establishing emotional rapport with others.

One of the goals of trauma-informed training to healthcare professionals is to improve recognition of trauma exposure and the associated risk of psychological distress and other negative social and health-related outcomes. The goal, however, is not to teach healthcare professionals that only patients with a history of trauma would benefit from the provision of trauma-informed care, but rather to teach these professionals that all patients would benefit from the provision of trauma-informed care [15]. MHPs can also provide education on the psychosocial and neurobiological consequences of trauma. Prevalence rates of trauma exposure and psychological distress within the general population as well as among the reproductive medicine patient population should be reviewed with staff and clinicians to illustrate the pervasiveness, severity, and consequences of psychological distress. MHPs may also consider highlighting the cumulative nature of trauma and the correlations between exposure to trauma and levels of somatization, anxiety/depression, sense of safety, and negative health consequences [15].

Some of the consequences of trauma exposure and psychological distress include coping strategies (e.g., substance use, dysfunctional eating behaviors, hypervigilance, high need for validation) which may be concerning to medical teams and others in the patient's life. MHPs can clarify that trauma-exposed or otherwise distressed individuals may cope with their distress in maladaptive ways which can also be described as survival techniques that helped the patient endure and cope with trauma. It is important for staff and medical teams to also recognize that the symptoms and consequences of trauma exposure and/or psychological distress can impact patients' adherence to medical treatment(s) due to avoidant behaviors, cognitive impairments, heightened emotional arousal to perceived loss of control, and fear of vulnerability in the presence of authority figures, such as medical professionals [16].

The interpersonal consequences of trauma exposure and psychological distress are also important to review with reproductive medicine clinic staff as they can impact patient-healthcare professional interactions. Reproductive medicine patients with psychological distress are faced with navigating the substantial stressors associated with reproductive treatment(s) while also managing their underlying mental health. Such individuals may also be experiencing new traumas and/or distress tied to their diagnosis of infertility and/or participation in assisted reproduction. When combined, these factors can lead to miscommunications and misperceptions between patients and healthcare professionals. For example, posttraumatic stress disorder alters the neurocognitive pathways that process and interpret social interactions [17]. Individuals with PTSD may be more likely to perceive innocuous interpersonal exchanges as being rejecting. Relationships with power differentials, such as the ones between patients and healthcare professionals, may seem threatening to individuals with PTSD [18, 19]. Trust in authority figures, such as medical professionals and MHPs, can erode following the experience of trauma(s). Patients who feel unsafe in the presence of authority figures or in situations wherein they are experiencing a loss of sense of control (e.g., infertility) may cope by passively complying, avoiding treatment, becoming contentious toward their healthcare professionals/staff, attempting to gain control of all aspects of treatment, and/or combativeness. Cultivating the ability to view patients' behaviors through a lens of distress and trauma may help increase empathy toward individuals who have experienced trauma [20]. With this lens, patients are no longer seen as "needy" or "difficult" but rather as people who are likely traumatized by past life experiences, struggling to cope with their current experience of infertility, scared about their future fertility, and in need of support and understanding. MHPs can facilitate conversations among clinic staff and healthcare professionals regarding balancing trauma-informed healthcare with holding patients accountable for unacceptable behaviors, such as verbal abuse of staff and/or healthcare professionals [17]. For example, fertility clinics should consider setting clear expectations regarding unacceptable patient behaviors at the initiation of treatment.

To deepen the trauma knowledge of reproductive medicine professionals and staff, MHPs can discuss the overlap between infertility and trauma. One's assumptions about themselves, others, and the world around them can be shattered in response to reproductive challenges and/or traumatic events [21]. The psychological sequelae of infertility and PTSD share various affective components, such as shame, guilt, loss of sense of control, fear, and sense of failure [22]. Individuals diagnosed with PTSD and/or infertility tend to possess negative perceptions of themselves and engage in self-blaming behavior. Disruptions in interpersonal relations are common subsequent to trauma as well as infertility diagnosis. The coping mechanisms of some reproductive medicine patients can also mirror that of coping skills utilized by individuals exposed to trauma(s) [21]. The invasive nature of most fertility tests and interventions may also reactivate PTSD symptoms from previous traumas [23].

While fraught with emotional distress, infertility and other difficult reproductive experiences are also an opportunity for personal growth [24, 25]. MHPs offering educational workshops on trauma-informed care to reproductive medicine clinics may consider discussing the concept of posttraumatic growth. Posttraumatic growth describes the phenomenon wherein people who have been exposed to trauma are able to eventually experience growth in resiliency, relationships, self-worth, meaning in their life, and other ways as a result of surviving and coping following the trauma [26]. Educating reproductive medicine teams about the possibility of posttraumatic growth can help provide a more balanced view of trauma and speaks to the incredible resilience demonstrated by some trauma-exposed individuals. It should be noted that not all trauma-exposed individuals experience posttraumatic growth and healthcare professionals should not shame patients who do not report such growth nor should they invalidate patients' experiences of pain by suggesting that they should stop feeling/thinking/talking about their trauma and instead focus on growth or resilience.

Modifications of Clinic Procedures, Operations, and Policies

The policies, procedures, and practices of healthcare systems can re-traumatize patients and reinforce harmful exclusionary practices. [27, 28]. There are a number of ways in which MHPs can aid in the removal of such practices. First, MHP provision of educational training sessions should be inclusive of the various types and dimensions of trauma as lack of awareness of the diverse nature of trauma can lead to the traumatization/re-traumatization of patients. For example, although many might initially think of interpersonal violence (e.g., physical/sexual assault) when discussing trauma and the development of PTSD or distress; trauma can also be experienced non-interpersonally (e.g., being trapped in a burning building, receiving a life altering medical diagnosis such as infertility), collectively (e.g., witnessing the events of 9/11 through media/television, attending the funeral of a woman who died during childbirth), and intergenerationally (e.g., children of Holocaust survivors). Trainings by MHPs should include education that healthcare professionals ought not to make personal judgments about whether trauma described by patients "count" as being traumatic because the patient's perception of their experience is of utmost importance in guiding their care.

The cultural context of trauma should also not be overlooked nor should the implicit biases of healthcare professionals (including MHPs). It is known that heteronormativity/ homophobia, cisnormativity/transphobia, sexism, racism, ableism, and other factors influence the frequency and severity of traumatic events experienced by various populations [29, 30]. Despite this fact, insufficient attention is paid to the ways in which exclusionary policies/practices and microaggressions can lead to the development, maintenance, and exacerbation of psychological distress and PTSD [20]. Reproductive medicine staff and healthcare professionals frequently interact with patients who have at least one identity that is historically disadvantaged and/or oppressed, such as women and LGBTQ+ identified patients. Just like all members of any society, reproductive clinic members may also hold implicit biases related to patients who differ from them in some way (e.g., socioeconomic status, gender identity, race/ethnicity, sexual orientation, etc.). As a result, MHPs should provide education on historic and current societal factors that shape the experiences of trauma while also helping clinic team members identify and correct implicit biases they may have, given that such biases can negatively affect the provision and receipt of patient care [31].

In addition, the assumption of heterosexuality and cisgender identity continues to exist within many reproductive medicine clinics. For example, there is often limited LGBTQ+ content on reproductive medicine clinics' websites [32]. Many LGBTQ+ patients also find their reproductive medicine clinics' paperwork to be non-inclusive of sexual minority couples [28]. Treatment can also be perceived as exclusionary if reproductive medicine teams do not include gender neutral and/or LGBTQ+ inclusionary language on clinic forms (e.g., intake forms describe partners as "wife" and "husband," instructions about sexual abstinence include only heterosexual intercourse, no options are provided to list patient pronouns).

MHPs can aid in the identification and removal of oppressive social views within fertility clinics by reviewing reproductive medicine clinics' paperwork, advertisements, and physical spaces to ensure that inclusivity, evidence of acceptance and safety, and representation of various groups of individuals are conveyed throughout the clinic. If desired, formal assessment of reproductive medicine patient experiences of inclusion and safety can be conducted by qualified MHPs and such evaluations can serve as a guide for ongoing need for training related to culturally sensitive trauma-informed care in the provision of patient care.

When it comes to the implementation of culturally sensitive trauma-informed care, MHPs must also look within their own professions and question whether cultural contexts and intersectional identities were taken into consideration upon developing the current evidence-based treatments for psychological distress including PTSD [33]. MHPs have a responsibility to learn about and provide culturally modified treatments to their patients. Specifically, MHPs must familiarize themselves with when and how to incorporate patients' migration history, acculturation process, value conflicts, spirituality/faith, interpersonal roles, and other layers of identities into existing psychotherapies. MHPs must also be transparent with patients regarding any lack of cultural competency in the provision of care to diverse patients and seek out any additional training.

There is a growing body of literature on culturally modified cognitive behavioral therapy for LGBTQ+ individuals, Latinas, and African Americans (see [33, 34] for review). There are many benefits to utilizing culturally modified psychotherapies including increased efficacy of treatment and higher patient satisfaction [34–36]. Trainings and certification on culturally modified psychotherapies can be found by utilizing online search engines and through requests to the MHP's respective national or state professional society.

Secondary Trauma

MHPs and other healthcare professionals who work with patients undergoing reproductive medical care may find the work both rewarding and emotionally challenging at times. Healthcare professionals (including MHPs) are vulnerable to secondary or vicarious trauma due to being exposed to patients' reports of trauma and/or witnessing patients experiencing trauma. The rates of secondary trauma among reproductive medicine healthcare professionals and staff are unknown. However, it is undeniable that reproductive medicine heathcare professionals and staff are exposed to patients' traumas due to the often traumatic nature of infertility diagnoses as well as the occurrences of reproductive losses. To help mitigate the negative effects of secondary trauma on healthcare professionals' professional and personal lives, MHPs with appropriate knowledge and training in secondary trauma can offer workshops to reproductive medicine clinics to educate medical teams about secondary trauma, provide relevant coping strategies, and provide information about how team members can obtain formal psychological support if needed.

The physical, emotional, cognitive, and behavioral symptoms of secondary traumatic stress mirror those of PTSD (guilt, helplessness, difficulties concentrating, sleep disturbance, hypervigilance, social withdrawal, increased heart rate). Secondary trauma is also linked to burnout and compassion fatigue among healthcare professionals. When experienced for extended periods of time, secondary traumatic stress leads to a decline in healthcare professionals' efficacy [37]. It is important for reproductive medicine staff and healthcare professionals to recognize the ways in which secondary trauma can impact their personal and professional lives. MHPs can review individual and organizational strategies aimed at preventing/reducing secondary trauma among healthcare professionals during clinic-wide trainings. It may be helpful for MHPs to discuss when and how fertility staff/healthcare professionals should seek professional health for their secondary trauma, such as through an employee assistance program or by meeting with a psychotherapist who specializes in caring for healthcare professionals and frontline employees.

It is important for clinic members to be aware that some medical professionals and staff experience both secondary trauma from their professional duties as well as PTSD or other pre-existing psychological conditions from their personal histories.

The fact that one's colleagues may be experiencing PTSD and its sequelae may not readily come to mind but should be discussed by MHPs who provide trauma-informed care training. Doing so can encourage trauma-informed changes on an organizational level and help cultivate compassion and sensitivity between colleagues [20]. In fact, research on trauma-informed workplaces found that professionals who undergo trauma-informed care training report greater sense of comradery and empathy for their colleagues [38].

Referrals to Mental Health Services

While psychological distress secondary to infertility and assisted reproductive technologies is common, the vast majority of men and women (>75%) undergoing fertility treatment in one study reported not having been provided with information on mental health services from their clinics. Patients in the same study who experienced significant psychological symptoms were also no more likely to receive referrals to mental health treatment from their fertility treatment team. Providing referrals to appropriate resources is an important aspect of trauma-informed care as it supports patient empowerment and helps cultivate trustworthiness [39].

MHPs can help increase reproductive medicine clinics' awareness of mental health referral options by providing names of MHPs with competency in the provision of trauma-informed care. MHPs can also demonstrate ways in which clinic staff and healthcare professionals can recommend mental health referrals to patients while simultaneously respecting patient autonomy and destigmatizing receipt of mental health support. MHPs can model the normalization of participation in mental health care when providing referrals to patients. For example, staff and healthcare professionals may choose to say, "Given how stressful fertility treatment can be, we always provide mental health resources to our patients. Many of our patients find it helpful to have additional support during this time." Given that reproductive challenges are often shared within a dyad, referrals to couple's counseling may be beneficial to aid in improved communication and coping.

Regarding medication management of psychological distress, it is not uncommon for patients undergoing assisted reproduction to stop utilizing their psychotropic medication(s) in preparation for pregnancy [40]. Self-discontinuation of psychotropic medications during fertility treatment is associated with recurrence of mental illness [40]. Patients who have self-discontinued their psychotropic medication(s) and/or have untreated or under-treated symptoms of a psychiatric disorder(s) may find it beneficial to meet with a reproductive psychiatrist to fully discuss the risk–benefit ratio of taking psychotropic medications during hormonal transitions, such as undergoing fertility treatment. Reproductive psychiatry often plays an integral role in the management of mental health conditions during fertility treatment, pregnancy, and postpartum. Psychotropic medications are frequently prescribed to reduce mood lability and risk of postpartum psychosis [41]. Patients exhibiting or reporting any mental health condition(s) of severe or moderately severe intensity should be referred to both reproductive psychiatry and psychotherapy. Patients with a history of significant hormonal sensitivities, such as premenstrual dysphoric disorder, may also benefit from establishing care with a psychotherapist and reproductive psychiatrist as they embark on fertility treatment.

It is important to consider that some reproductive medicine patients may not have an interest in or feel comfortable engaging in individual mental health treatment. As a result, patients should be provided various mental health and support options. For instance, to help connect patients with their peers, which is a tenet of trauma-informed care, healthcare professionals and staff can direct patients to trauma and/or fertility-related support groups led by trained peer supporters. When possible, specific information regarding the focus of the peer-led groups (e.g., general trauma, reproductive trauma, infertility following cancer, etc.) should be provided so that patients can make informed choices about their participation in mental health care.

Trauma-Informed Care in Gate-Keeping Role

MHPs fulfill several roles, such as psychotherapist, consultant, and, for those who provide third-party reproduction evaluative services, gate-keeper. Per the guidelines set forth by the American Society for Reproductive Medicine ([42]), gamete donors and gestational carrier candidates undergo a psychological evaluation prior to the initiation of fertility-related medical treatment. During these psychological evaluations, trauma inquiries are indicated and conducted (in detail, if pertinent to candidacy). The information gleaned from the clinical interview and psychological test results of gamete donors and gestational carriers may disqualify candidates from participating in those roles. Gamete donors and surrogacy candidates may find it traumatizing or re-traumatizing to undergo trauma inquiry and/or be deemed ineligible to be a gamete donor or gestational carrier. They may find the assessment process to be reminiscent of previous interpersonal betrayals, losses of control, or abuses of power that they may have endured [43]. Currently, there are no known models of trauma-informed assessment of gamete donors and gestational carriers specifically; however, the principles of trauma-informed care can be readily applied.

In the context of third-party reproduction, MHPs often serve various roles. For the purposes of transparency and establishing trust with patients, it is vital that MHPs clarify their specific roles when working with gamete donors, gestational carriers, and intended parents/recipients. All involved parties should be aware if and when they are being psychologically evaluated. This information and the content of psychological appointments (e.g., donors will be asked about their developmental, trauma, and substance use histories) should be clearly written in consent forms and verbally discussed with patients. Assessors should also strive to convey genuine empathy (verbal and/or non-verbal) toward examinees while also maintaining objectivity [44]. In order to develop such skills, MHPs should consider undergoing further training and/or consulting with colleagues to ensure impartiality. Another way to integrate trauma-informed care into the third-party reproduction psychological evaluations is to ensure that the examiner is fully trained and competent in utilizing assessment instruments. Lack of appropriate training and supervision in the administration and interpretations of psychological assessment instruments may lead to the unnecessary disqualification or inappropriate acceptance of gamete donors/gestational carriers.

Embedded and Consultative MHPs

It is well-documented that the integration of qualified MHPs into primary care clinics optimizes patient outcomes and staff well-being [45]. Similarly, the embedment of MHPs in fertility clinics is considered best practice [46]. Fertility patients who have access to an onsite MHP perceive their overall treatment experience to be more positive [47]. However, the vast majority of reproductive medicine clinics do not have embedded MHPs and, instead, seek consultative relationships with external MHPs.

Embedded MHPs support their colleagues and patients by providing curbside consultations regarding patient care and accepting "warm hand-offs" (the transfer of care between healthcare team members) from other healthcare professionals. The conveniences and familiarities associated with receiving care from an embedded MHP may empower patients to engage in mental health care. Patients referred to an embedded MHP will likely be acquainted with the scheduling procedures at their clinic and may be able to schedule their mental health and medical appointments with one phone call. In addition, the clinic's financial counseling department may be able to screen patients' mental health benefits, which is perceived by patients as a barrier to receiving mental health care. Patients who feel hesitant or uncomfortable rehashing the details of their reproductive and trauma histories with a new MHP may prefer to meet with embedded MHPs, who typically have full access to their patients' electronic medical records.

Conversely, it is possible that some patients associate their reproductive medicine clinic and its team members with various traumatic events. As a result, returning to the clinic to receive care from an embedded MHP could potentially re-traumatize some patients. Similarly, patients who lack trust in or have had negative interactions with one or more team members at a reproductive medicine clinic may prefer to meet with an external MHP. It is also possible that some patients may feel like they can speak more freely about their reproductive treatment experiences when working with an MHP who is not employed by their clinic.

Conclusions

MHPs have contributed their unique perspectives and services to the field of reproductive endocrinology for multiple decades. Their involvement is instrumental to patient care as well as the well-being of healthcare professionals and staff [48]. As fertility counseling continues to grow and evolve, there is need for research in and practice modifications based on trauma-informed care specifically within the realm of infertility and assisted reproduction.

References

1. Boivin J, Gameiro S. Evolution of psychology and counseling in infertility. Fertil Steril. 2015;104:251–9.
2. Domar AD, Zuttermeister PC, Friedman R. The psychological impact of infertility: a comparison with patients with other medical conditions. J Psychosom Obstet Gynecol. 1993;14:45–52.
3. Lawson AK, Klock SC, Pavone ME, Hirshfeld-Cytron J, Smith KN, Kazer RR. Prospective study of depression and anxiety in female fertility preservation and infertility patients. Fertil Steril. 2014;102:1377–84.
4. Practice Committee of the American Society for Reproductive Medicine, Practice Committee of the Society for Assisted Reproductive Technology. Minimum standards for practices offering assisted reproductive technologies: a committee opinion. Fertil Steril. 2021;115:578–82.
5. Leeners B, Tschudin S, Wischmann T, Kalaitzopoulos DR. Sexual dysfunction and disorders as a consequence of infertility: a systematic review and meta-analysis. Hum Reprod Update. 2023;29(1):95–125. https://doi.org/10.1093/humupd/dmac030. PMID: 35900268.
6. Kolte AM, Olsen LR, Mikkelsen EM, Christiansen OB, Nielsen HS. Depression and emotional stress is highly prevalent among women with recurrent pregnancy loss. Hum Reprod. 2015;30(4):777–82. https://doi.org/10.1093/humrep/dev014. Epub 2015 Feb 5. PMID: 25662810; PMCID: PMC4359400.
7. Montmasson H, Bertrand P, Perrotin F, El-Hage W. Predictors of postpartum post-traumatic stress disorder in primiparous mothers. J Gynecol Obstet Biol Reprod. 2012;41:553–60.
8. Roozitalab S, Rahimzadeh M, Mirmajidi SR, Ataee M, Saeieh SE. The relationship between infertility, stress, and quality of life with posttraumatic stress disorder in infertile women. J Reprod Infertil. 2021;22:282.
9. Committee P. Guidance on qualifications for fertility counselors: a committee opinion. Fertil Steril. 2021;115:1411–5.
10. Lewis-O'Connor A, Warren A, Lee JV, Levy-Carrick N, Grossman S, Chadwick M, Stoklosa H, Rittenberg E. The state of the science on trauma inquiry. Womens Health. 2019;15:15.
11. Reeves E. A synthesis of the literature on trauma-informed care. Issues Ment Health Nurs. 2015;36:698–709.
12. Felitti VJ, Anda RF, Nordenberg D, et al. Relationship of childhood abuse and household dysfunction to many of the leading causes of death in adults: the adverse childhood experiences (ACE) study. Am J Prev Med. 1998;14(4):245–58. https://doi.org/10.1016/S0749-3797(98)00017-8.
13. Hoffman J, Ben-Zion Z, Arévalo A, Duek O, Greene T, Hall BJ, Harpaz-Rotem I, Liddell B, Locher C, Morina N, Nickerson A, Pfaltz MC, Schick M, Schnyder U, Seedat S, Shatri F, Sit HF, von Känel R, Spiller TR. Mapping the availability of translated versions of posttraumatic stress disorder screening questionnaires for adults: a scoping review. Eur J Psychotraumatol. 2022;13(2):2143019. https://doi.org/10.1080/20008066.2022.2143019.

14. Lotzin A, Buth S, Sehner S, Hiller P, Martens MS, Pawils S, Metzner F, Read J, Härter M, Schäfer I. "Learning how to ask": effectiveness of a training for trauma inquiry and response in substance use disorder healthcare professionals. Psychol Trauma Theory Res Pract Policy. 2018;10:229.
15. Lathan EC, Selwyn CN, Langhinrichsen-Rohling J. The "3 Es" of trauma-informed care in a federally qualified health center: Traumatic Event- and Experience-related predictors of physical and mental health Effects among female patients. J Comm Psychol. 2021;49(2):703–24. https://doi.org/10.1002/jcop.22488.
16. Hayes JP, VanElzakker MB, Shin LM. Emotion and cognition interactions in PTSD: a review of neurocognitive and neuroimaging studies. Front Integr Neurosci. 2012;6:89.
17. Taft CT, Creech SK, Murphy CM. Anger and aggression in PTSD. Curr Opin Psychol. 2017;14:67–71.
18. Francis East J, Roll SJ. Women, poverty, and trauma: an empowerment practice approach. Soc Work. 2015;60:279–86.
19. Knight C. Trauma-informed social work practice: practice considerations and challenges. Clin Soc Work J. 2015;43:25–37.
20. Sweeney A, Filson B, Kennedy A, Collinson L, Gillard S. A paradigm shift: relationships in trauma-informed mental health services. BJPsych Adv. 2018;24:319–33.
21. Jaffe J. Reproductive trauma and PTSD: on the battlefield of fertility counseling. In: Fertility counseling: clinical guide; 2022. p. 204–11.
22. Heim E, Karatzias T, Maercker A. Cultural concepts of distress and complex PTSD: future directions for research and treatment. Clin Psychol Rev. 2022;93:102143.
23. Covington L. Trauma and its impact on reproduction and sexuality. In: Psychological and medical perspectives on fertility care and sexual health; 2022. p. 173–87.
24. Kong L, Fang M, Ma T, Li G, Yang F, Meng Q, Li Y, Li P. Positive affect mediates the relationships between resilience, social support and posttraumatic growth of women with infertility. Psychol Health Med. 2018;23:707–16.
25. Paul MS, Berger R, Berlow N, Rovner-Ferguson H, Figlerski L, Gardner S, Malave AF. Posttraumatic growth and social support in individuals with infertility. Hum Reprod. 2010;25:133–41.
26. Tedeschi RG, Calhoun LG. The posttraumatic growth inventory: measuring the positive legacy of trauma. J Trauma Stress. 1996;9:455–71.
27. Grossman S, Cooper Z, Buxton H, Hendrickson S, Lewis-O'Connor A, Stevens J, Wong LY, Bonne S. Trauma-informed care: recognizing and resisting re-traumatization in health care. TASCO. 2021;6:e000815.
28. Ortis C. Queering fertility: experiences of queer/lesbian people undergoing fertility treatment in a heteronormative society. Petaluma, CA: University of Northern California; 2019.
29. Asnaani A, Hall-Clark B. Recent developments in understanding ethnocultural and race differences in trauma exposure and PTSD. Curr Opin Psychol. 2017;14:96–101.
30. Russell ST, Fish JN. Mental health in lesbian, gay, bisexual, and transgender (LGBT) youth. Annu Rev Clin Psychol. 2016;12:465–87.
31. Vela MB, Erondu AI, Smith NA, Peek ME, Woodruff JN, Chin MH. Eliminating explicit and implicit biases in health care: evidence and research needs. Annu Rev Public Health. 2022;43:477–501.
32. Wu HY, Yin O, Monseur B, Selter J, Collins LJ, Lau BD, Christianson MS. Lesbian, gay, bisexual, transgender content on reproductive endocrinology and infertility clinic websites. Fertil Steril. 2017;108:183–91.
33. Bryant-Davis T. The cultural context of trauma recovery: considering the posttraumatic stress disorder practice guideline and intersectionality. Psychotherapy. 2019;56:400–8.
34. Anik E, West RM, Cardno AG, Mir G. Culturally adapted psychotherapies for depressed adults: a systematic review and meta-analysis. J Affect Disord. 2021;278:296–310.

35. Hwang WC, Myers HF, Chiu E, Mak E, Butner JE, Fujimoto K, Wood JJ, Miranda J. Culturally adapted cognitive-behavioral therapy for Chinese Americans with depression: a randomized controlled trial. Psychiatr Serv. 2015;66:1035–42.
36. Ponting C, Mahrer NE, Zelcer H, Dunkel Schetter C, Chavira DA. Psychological interventions for depression and anxiety in pregnant Latina and black women in the United States: a systematic review. Clin Psychol Psychother. 2020;27:249–65.
37. Jordan K. Trauma-informed counseling supervision: something every counselor should know about. Asia Pac J Counsel Psychother. 2018;9:127–42.
38. Damian AJ, Gallo J, Leaf P, Mendelson T. Organizational and provider level factors in implementation of trauma-informed care after a city-wide training: an explanatory mixed methods assessment. BMC Health Serv Res. 2017;17:1–10.
39. Pasch LA, Holley SR, Bleil ME, Shehab D, Katz PP, Adler NE. Addressing the needs of fertility treatment patients and their partners: are they informed of and do they receive mental health services? Fertil Steril. 2016;106:209–15.
40. Freeman MP, Lee H, Savella GM, Sosinsky AZ, Marfurt SP, Murphy SK, Cohen LS. Predictors of depressive relapse in women undergoing infertility treatment. J Womens Health. 2018;27:1408–14.
41. Sharma V, Sharma P, Sharma S. Managing bipolar disorder during pregnancy and the postpartum period: a critical review of current practice. Expert Rev Neurother. 2020;20:373–83.
42. Practice Committee of the American Society for Reproductive Medicine, Practice Committee of the Society for Assisted Reproductive Technology. Recommendations for gamete and embryo donation: a committee opinion. Fertil Steril. 2013;99:47–62.
43. Dalenberg CJ, Straus E, Ardill M. Forensic psychology in the context of trauma. In: APA handbook of trauma psychology: trauma practice; 2017. p. 543–63.
44. Goldenson J, Brodsky SL, Perlin ML. Trauma-informed forensic mental health assessment: Practical implications, ethical tensions, and alignment with therapeutic jurisprudence principles. Psychology, Public Policy, and Law, 2020;28(2), 226.
45. Prom MC, Canelos V, Fernandez PJ, Gergen Barnett K, Gordon CM, Pace CA, Ng LC. Implementation of integrated behavioral health care in a large medical center: benefits, challenges, and recommendations. J Behav Health Serv Res. 2021;48:346–62.
46. Sax MR, Lawson AK. Emotional support for infertility patients: Integrating mental health professionals in the fertility care team. Women. 2022;2:68–75. https://doi.org/10.3390/women2010008.
47. Shandley LM, Hipp HS, Anderson-Bialis J, Anderson-Bialis D, Boulet SL, McKenzie LJ, Kawwass JF. Patient-centered care: factors associated with reporting a positive experience at United States fertility clinics. Fertil Steril. 2020;113:797–810.
48. Facchin F, Leone D, Tamanza G, Costa M, Sulpizio P, Canzi E, Vegni E. Working with infertile couples seeking assisted reproduction: an interpretative phenomenological study with infertility care providers. Front Psychol. 2020;17:11.

Chapter 10
Special Considerations for Military Personnel, Veterans, and First Responders

Erika L. Kelley and Angela Lawson

Introduction

Several chapters in this book address trauma-informed care for specific populations. An additional population that should be considered within the Reproductive Endocrinology and Infertility (REI) setting are active-duty military service members and Veterans as well as First Responders (e.g., law enforcement personnel, firefighters, paramedics, emergency medical technicians, search and rescue personnel, 911/dispatch, emergency department personnel, etc.), for several reasons. Perhaps the most salient reason is the repeated exposure to experiencing and/or witnessing potentially traumatic events such as war, combat, physical and sexual violence, death or serious injury, and other threats to their personal well-being which are often part of their work experiences. Although the Adverse Childhood Events (ACEs) study finds that many individuals in the USA will experience one or more traumatic experiences prior to reaching adulthood [1], and many adults will experience additional traumatic experiences throughout the remainder of their lives [2], military personnel and First Responders experience these types of traumatic events on an even more frequent basis [3]. As a result of these cumulative exposures, military personnel and First Responders have a greater prevalence of

E. L. Kelley
Division of Behavioral Medicine, Department of OB/GYN, University Hospitals Cleveland Medical Center, Cleveland, OH, USA

Department of Reproductive Biology, School of Medicine, The Urology Institute, Case Western Reserve University, Cleveland, OH, USA

MacDonald Women's Hospital, Cleveland, OH, USA
e-mail: Erika.Kelley@UHhospitals.org

A. Lawson (✉)
Obstetrics and Gynecology, Northwestern Medicine, Chicago, IL, USA
e-mail: alawsonphd@gmail.com

A. Lawson, A. Swanson (eds.), *Trauma-Informed Reproductive Healthcare*,
https://doi.org/10.1007/978-3-031-67474-7_10

Posttraumatic Stress Disorder (PTSD), depression, and suicide than the general population with female military personnel and First Responders often (but not always) being at greater risk of the development of PTSD in part due to their greater risk of work-related sexual victimization [4–9]. For example, The Wave 3 National Epidemiologic Survey on Alcohol and Related Conditions (NESARC-III) [10] found an age- and race- adjusted lifetime prevalence of PTSD of 13.4% for women Veterans and 7.7% for men Veterans, compared with 8.0% in women civilians and 3.4% in men civilians. Estimates of lifetime PTSD prevalence are up to 22% in EMT/paramedics and up to 32% in firefighters [11]. Despite this higher risk for the development of PTSD, many active-duty military personnel, Veterans, and First Responders underreport their experiences due to the stigma associated with psychiatric diagnoses and some traumatic events, and the often realistic concern that a mental health diagnosis will negatively affect their careers in these occupations [12–14].

Underreporting of trauma is especially prominent in military members and First Responders who experience sexual assault or other sexual victimization from those to whom they are providing aid and/or from fellow First Responders or military personnel [15–18]. Military sexual trauma (MST) is the term used by the U.S. Department of Veterans Affairs to describe sexual assault (involving any level of unwanted sexual activity) or threatening sexual harassment that occurs during military service. Like active-duty military personnel, many First Responders work in environments with hierarchical structures, some may work non-traditional hours which require them to work 24 hour or longer shifts and sleep in close proximity to the individual(s) who has victimized them (e.g., firehouses), and like military personnel, many are required to report their experiences of victimization up a chain of command, which may include individuals who are friends of the perpetrator or who are unsupportive of allegations of victimization. Furthermore, concerns related to lack of support in reporting and confidentiality of reporting leading to fear of retaliation including non-support during future work-related life or death situations for First Responders and military personnel alike, or other career consequences such as not receiving an expected promotion, discharge from service, or an unanticipated relocation, may serve as barriers to disclosure [17–19].

Cumulative Trauma Exposure and Need for Trauma-Informed Care

The cumulative exposure to traumas such as those experienced by military personnel and First Responders not only increases the risk of the development of PTSD but the exposure to trauma also increases their risk of other health and psychosocial problems such as infertility [1, 20–22]. It may also result in increased distress due to a loss of feelings of control during the receipt of healthcare, particularly healthcare which involves physical exams such as pelvic exams or other care that risks re-traumatizing patients. Trauma-informed care is a person-centered, recovery-oriented, empowerment focused delivery of medical care. In practice, trauma-informed care comes from a place of understanding of the prevalence and health and other negative effects of trauma, recognizes trauma sequalae, and responds to patients' needs in ways that avoid re-traumatization and promote healing [23]. Several studies highlight the importance of the provision of trauma-informed care (including the presence of an integrated health psychologist) during primary care and reproductive care in aiding the development of medical trust, decreasing re-traumatization, increasing feelings of control, and increasing feelings of safety for military personnel (see, e.g., [24, 25]). Although limited research has been conducted which examines the application of trauma-informed care for First Responders, it appears likely that given their similarities to military personnel in terms of cumulative trauma exposure (and risk of physical and/or sexual assault in particular) as well as organizational structures and cultures, the provision of trauma-informed care would be similarly effective in promoting healing and reducing harm in this population.

The provision of trauma-informed healthcare requires that healthcare professionals screen patients for histories of trauma and trauma sequalae in order to understand the shared and unique medical and other correlates of the patient's trauma experience(s). Research shows, however, that healthcare professionals, including reproductive healthcare professionals, do not adequately screen patients for history of trauma(s) [26]. In addition, research indicates that military service is underassessed by healthcare professionals, and healthcare professionals commonly report discomfort with assessing for military service history and with addressing conditions prevalent among Veterans [27, 28]. Given the prevalence of trauma exposure in the general population and the high risk of symptoms of PTSD and increased risk of physical/sexual assault and harassment in military personnel and First Responders, it could be easily argued that even in the absence of appropriate screening, all patients should be provided with trauma-informed care. However, it is important again to note that there are shared and unique sequalae to different kinds of trauma. For example, someone involved in a traumatic automobile accident may experience distressing psychological or physiological arousal when exposed to stimuli that remind them of the accident (e.g., hearing car horns, seeing car accidents, and/or riding in a car) whereas someone who has been sexually assaulted may experience distress upon exposure to different stimuli (e.g., pelvic and other physical exams, intimacy, threats to their physical or sexual safety). Thus, without appropriate screening of the unique trauma(s) experienced by patients, it is not possible to provide adequate trauma-informed care. Healthcare professionals should not rely on patients voluntarily disclosing their experiences of trauma or try to guess which patient has experienced trauma. Instead, healthcare professionals should sensitively ask patients, using behaviorally specific language when possible, about such experiences and ask all patients about military service, Veteran status, and First Responder occupational status. It is important to ask about past, current, and future intended service; if asking about only current occupational status when gathering a patient's sociodemographic information, important information can be missed. Given stereotypes of military personnel and First Responders as stoic and resilient, assumptions should also never be made about who has or has not been exposed to trauma as these stereotypes are unreliable [14, 29].

Trauma-Informed Reproductive Care Considerations for Military Personnel and First Responders

Unlike First Responders whose medical insurance benefits may cover them for fertility treatments and who use public and private medical centers for the majority of their general medical care, at the time of writing this chapter, some fertility services for military families are not covered by the Veterans Affairs (VA) medical benefits package within the VA health care systems. Furthermore, many military personnel receive the large majority of their health care from VA health care settings (the largest integrated health care system in the USA). In addition to the potential need to seek fertility care outside of the VA health care system, there is also a notable portion of military personnel who primarily seek medical care outside of the VA health care system [30]. Due to the shared knowledge of the types of trauma military personnel may experience, receipt of healthcare within the VA health care system is likely to be more trauma-informed than healthcare in civilian medical systems and the transition to civilian medical care may result in anxiety related to how they will be perceived (e.g., stigmatized) and treated as trauma-survivors in these systems. As previously discussed, First Responders may also worry about experiencing stigmatization from healthcare professionals when disclosing their experience of trauma.

Military personnel and First Responders may also be exposed to unique experiences or factors that may affect reproductive health, such as environmental and occupational exposures (e.g., heat, smoke, radiation, and toxins), military or workplace sexual trauma, and combat or other physical injuries [31, 32]. As previously discussed, military personnel and First Responders are also at a higher risk for cumulative trauma exposure than the general public and may experience more frequent and/or unique types of traumatic event exposures (e.g., combat trauma, seeing badly injured or dead bodies). They may also experience these traumas within unique cultural settings, which discourage organizational reporting of traumatic events and their psychological impact as this may affect the individual's ability to serve or be promoted. As a result, they may experience unique trauma cues and reminders. It is also important to note that military personnel and First Responders may have concerns related to disclosing trauma experiences or mental health symptoms to their healthcare professionals for fear that such information will be documented in their medical records and will thereby negatively affect their careers. Healthcare professionals should therefore not assume that military or First Responder patients have no history of trauma or PTSD even if they deny such a history. During the assessment of trauma and mental health symptoms, the healthcare professional should acknowledge awareness of the potential difficulties in disclosing trauma or mental health concerns given the patient's occupation, discuss the limits of confidentiality and medical documentation, and offer referral information for mental health professionals and peer support programs (e.g., The National Alliance on Mental Illness, Frontline Professionals resources https://www.nami.org/Your-Journey/Frontline-Professionals). It is also important to clearly describe whether (and if so, how) mental health symptoms (such as PTSD) could affect their ability to engage in assisted reproductive technology or participation as a gamete donor or gestational carrier.

As noted above, successful trauma-informed care requires an empathic understanding of the specific population with whom an organization or individual is working. Notably, the specific era of service or specific role as a First Responder may be beneficial to understanding a patient. For example, experiences can vary across military Veteran eras, such as the specific combat equipment and techniques, combat medicine and protective gear available, physical location of the traumatic event(s), and the sociocultural context at the timing of a specific war, which can affect a Veteran's health [33]. Healthcare professionals who may interact with military personnel and First Responders would benefit from education around military and First Responder culture and experience. Clinic administrators can consider providing this specific education to staff as part of trauma-informed care training.

Consideration of trauma-informed care for military personnel and First Responders is not limited to only those personnel who are currently serving in these roles. For example, it is not uncommon for military personnel to engage in gamete cryopreservation prior to deployment in order to preserve the chance to have genetic children should they be injured during combat/war [34]. The decision to freeze gametes in these instances may therefore be associated with a different kind of anxiety than that typically seen in single patients who may primarily be concerned about not having a partner with whom to grow their family. Though both groups (single patients and those being deployed) may engage in gamete cryopreservation due to concerns about reduced chance of success in the context of delayed family building, military personnel are also likely anxious about their risk of serious injury (which could impair their fertility) and death. Care should be taken to support the emotional needs of military personnel and First Responders engaging in gamete preservation prior to deployment. Additionally, given the increased risk of death for active-duty military personnel and First Responders, counseling related to posthumous reproduction and gamete disposition preferences are vital for these patients and their partners [34]. Documentation of patient wishes with regard to gamete disposition may not only be beneficial when surviving loved ones return to discuss and/or utilize the deceased's cryopreserved gametes but also may serve as a reminder to engage in trauma-informed care with surviving loved ones [35].

Recommendations for Trauma-Informed Care with Military Personnel and First Responders

Some example recommendations for trauma-informed care with military and First Responder patients, which can be considered within clinic procedures and education to staff, include the following: asking about (and acknowledging) military and First Responder status, era of service, and occupation type or role; thanking them for their service; being sure to clarify documentation procedures, limits of confidentiality, and procedures related to releases of medical information to the patient prior to assessing trauma history; avoiding having them recount their trauma history multiple times; asking for consent before closing an office door and knocking before entering a room; modifying or asking for consent before doing relaxation exercises that include closed eyes; avoiding language such as "ordering" an examination or lab work and instead using "requesting" or "submitting a request"; avoiding exposing the patient to specimens obtained during D&Cs or other procedures; sensitivity to patient anxiety related to emergency procedures or miscarrying at home; treating all coworkers regardless of professional status with respect and without ordering them to complete tasks (e.g., politely request that they complete a needed task); and asking the patient about their specific triggers to help inform treatment planning [33]. In addition, some common examples of triggers for this population include sudden movements, being approached from behind, sitting with their back to the door/exit, hearing screams of pain, and loud noises (e.g., slamming a file cabinet shut). Additional recommendations for trauma-informed care can be found in Chap. 3 of this book for patients who have experienced sexual victimization and a summary of considerations for trauma-informed care for military personnel and First Responders can be found in Table 10.1. Clinic administrators may consider collaborations with Veteran's and First Responder service organizations to maximize care for patients. Furthermore, the US Department of Veterans Affairs (see www.va.gov) provides many educational and training resources regarding working with Veteran patients that may also be applicable to First Responders.

Conclusions

Active-duty military personnel, Veterans, and First Responders are at greater risk of the development of PTSD than the general population due to cumulative exposure to often life threatening or otherwise traumatic events over prolonged periods of time. The organizational culture of these occupations may limit the reporting of trauma experiences to employers and to healthcare professionals, result in re-victimization via retaliation or invalidation of the individual's experience, and may result in reduced engagement in mental health care to address trauma symptoms. Research supports the importance of the provision of trauma-informed medical care to military personnel and First Responders. Effective provision of trauma-informed

Table 10.1 Summary of considerations relevant to the provision of trauma-informed care (TIC) to active-duty military personnel, veterans, and first responders

TIC considerations	Risks to military personnel and first responders	TIC behaviors
Nature of trauma	• Frequent exposure • Cumulative effect of traumas • Witnessing trauma to others • Combat exposure • Toxin exposure • Life threatening events or contexts • Physical and/or sexual assault • Serious injury • Infertility due to trauma	• Thank patients for their service/work • Ask about: – Known trauma triggers – Era of service and role – Types of traumas experienced – Risk of future trauma (e.g., deployment)
Trauma sequelae	• Posttraumatic stress disorder • Suicidality • Substance use • Anxiety • Depression • Infertility • Negative health outcomes	• Screen for mental health symptoms • Discuss limits to confidentiality and patient concerns • Refer to mental health professionals • Refer to confidential peer support
Barriers to care	• Fear of disclosing trauma and psychological symptoms • Career concerns • Fear of retaliation • Harmful stereotypes • Failure to assess trauma triggers • Failure to provide TIC • Inadequate medical team knowledge of unique work-related experiences	• Discuss limits to confidentiality • Avoid reliance on stereotypes • Assess for trauma and occupation/service • Obtain training related to TIC in military and first responder populations • Avoid re-traumatization
Fertility concerns	• Gamete cryopreservation prior to deployment • Infertility due to trauma – Toxin exposure – Physical injury – Sexual assault – Death/injury of partner • Posthumous reproduction • Delayed family building	• Provide emotional support • Counsel and document gamete disposition wishes • Use TIC during posthumous reproduction cycles • Counsel for gamete cryopreservation

care requires that healthcare professionals understand patients' unique trauma experiences and triggers. As such, healthcare professionals should ask all patients about any history of military service (including era and combat exposure), work as a First Responder (including types of trauma exposures) and known trauma triggers. Awareness of and sensitivity to patients concerns about the medical documentation of trauma exposure and mental health symptoms coupled with appropriate referrals for confidential support are vital for creating a safe environment for military and First Responder patients. Finally, consideration of military personnel and First Responders' emotional needs related to gamete cryopreservation prior to deployment and posthumous reproduction is imperative in the provision of trauma-informed care.

References

1. Merrick MT, Ford DC, Ports KA, Guinn AS. Prevalence of adverse childhood experiences from the 2011-2014 behavioral risk factor surveillance system in 23 states. JAMA Pediatr. 2018;172(11):1038–44.
2. Ogle CM, Rubin DC, Berntsen D, Siegler IC. The frequency and impact of exposure to potentially traumatic events over the life course. Clin Psychol Sci. 2013;1(4):426–34.
3. Hartley TA, Violanti JM, Sarkisian K, Andrew ME, Burchfiel CM. PTSD symptoms among police officers: associations with frequency, recency, and types of traumatic events. Int J Emerg Ment Health. 2013;15:241–53.
4. Berger W, Coutinho ES, Figueira I, Marques-Portella C, Luz MP, Neylan TC, et al. Rescuers at risk: a systematic review and meta-regression analysis of the worldwide current prevalence and correlates of PTSD in rescue workers. Soc Psychiatry Psychiatr Epidemiol. 2012;47(6):1001–11.
5. Zinzow HM, Grubaugh AL, Monnier J, Suffoletta-Maierle S, Frueh BC. Trauma among female veterans: a critical review. Trauma Violence Abuse. 2007;8(4):384–400.
6. Judkins JL, Moore BA, Collette TL, Hale WJ, Peterson AL, Morissette SB. Incidence rates of posttraumatic stress disorder over a 17-year period in active duty military service members. J Trauma Stress. 2020;33(6):994–1006.
7. Petrie K, Milligan-Saville J, Gayed A, Deady M, Phelps A, Dell L, et al. Prevalence of PTSD and common mental disorders amongst ambulance personnel: a systematic review and meta-analysis. Soc Psychiatry Psychiatr Epidemiol. 2018;53(9):897–909.
8. Tatebe LC, Rajaram Siva N, Pekarek S, Liesen E, Wheeler A, Reese C, et al. Heroes in crisis: trauma centers should be screening for and intervening on posttraumatic stress in our emergency responders. J Trauma Acute Care Surg. 2020;89(1):132–9.
9. Hoell A, Kourmpeli E, Dressing H. Work-related posttraumatic stress disorder in paramedics in comparison to data from the general population of working age. A systematic review and meta-analysis. Front Public Health. 2023;11:1151248.
10. Lehavot K, Katon JG, Chen JA, Fortney JC, Simpson TL. Post-traumatic stress disorder by gender and veteran status. Am J Prev Med. 2018;54(1):e1–9.
11. Lewis-Schroeder NF, Kieran K, Murphy BL, Wolff JD, Robinson MA, Kaufman ML. Conceptualization, assessment, and treatment of traumatic stress in first responders: a review of critical issues. Harv Rev Psychiatry. 2018;26(4):216–27.
12. Marshall RE, Milligan-Saville J, Petrie K, Bryant RA, Mitchell PB, Harvey SB. Mental health screening amongst police officers: factors associated with under-reporting of symptoms. BMC Psychiatry. 2021;21(1):135.
13. Hom MA, Stanley IH, Schneider ME, Joiner TE Jr. A systematic review of help-seeking and mental health service utilization among military service members. Clin Psychol Rev. 2017;53:59–78.
14. Jones S, Agud K, McSweeney J. Barriers and facilitators to seeking mental health care among first responders: "removing the darkness". J Am Psychiatr Nurses Assoc. 2020;26(1):43–54.
15. Jahnke SA, Haddock CK, Jitnarin N, Kaipust CM, Hollerbach BS, Poston WSC. The prevalence and health impacts of frequent work discrimination and harassment among women firefighters in the US fire service. Biomed Res Int. 2019;2019:6740207.
16. Abbott I, Whitley GA. What are ambulance personnel experiences of sexual harassment and sexual assault in the workplace? A rapid evidence review. Int Emerg Nurs. 2023;71:101376.

17. Tosto SA. Prosecuting military sexual assault: the entanglement of military discourse and victim stereotypes in prosecutor case strategies. Fem Criminol. 2023;18(5):459–89.
18. Williams MT, Bartlett A, Zare M, Custer N, Osman M. Sexual harassment and abuse in law enforcement: best practices for creating safety for female officers. Police J. 2022;97:205.
19. Perket S, McQueeney K. Harassment, discrimination, and assault: the unseen crisis in fire service professions. J Student Res. 2022;11(4):1–14.
20. Ryan GL, Mengeling MA, Booth BM, Torner JC, Syrop CH, Sadler AG. Voluntary and involuntary childlessness in female veterans: associations with sexual assault. Fertil Steril. 2014;102(2):539–47.
21. Serrano-Ibanez ER, Corras T, Del Prado M, Diz J, Varela C. Psychological variables associated with post-traumatic stress disorder in firefighters: a systematic review. Trauma Violence Abuse. 2023;24(4):2049–66.
22. Karam EG, Friedman MJ, Hill ED, Kessler RC, McLaughlin KA, Petukhova M, et al. Cumulative traumas and risk thresholds: 12-month PTSD in the world mental health (WMH) surveys. Depress Anxiety. 2014;31(2):130–42.
23. Kelly U, Boyd MA, Valente SM, Czekanski E. Trauma-informed care: keeping mental health settings safe for veterans. Issues Ment Health Nurs. 2014;35(6):413–9.
24. Gopisetty DD, Shaw JG, Gray C, Frayne S, Phibbs C, Shankar M. Veteran postpartum health: VA care team perspectives on care coordination, health equity, and trauma-informed care. Mil Med. 2022;188:e1563.
25. Carlson GC, Than CT, Rose D, Brunner J, Chanfreau-Coffinier C, Canelo IA, et al. What drives women Veterans' Trust in VA healthcare providers? Womens Health Issues. 2022;32(5):499–508.
26. Farrow VA, Bosch J, Crawford JN, Snead C, Schulkin J. Screening for history of childhood abuse: beliefs, practice patterns, and barriers among obstetrician-gynecologists. Womens Health Issues. 2018;28(6):559–68.
27. Vest BM, Kulak J, Hall VM, Homish GG. Addressing patients' veteran status: primary care providers' knowledge, comfort, and educational needs. Fam Med. 2018;50(6):455–9.
28. Miller KE, Finn JA, Newman E. Are communities ready? Assessing providers' practices, attitudes, and knowledge about military personnel. Prof Psychol Res Pract. 2014;45(6):398–404.
29. Mika-Lude KM, Degges-White S, Isawi D. Under fire: meta-dehumanization and burnout among first responders. J Employ Couns. 2023;60(3):144–58.
30. Nelson KM, Starkebaum GA, Reiber GE. Veterans using and uninsured veterans not using veterans affairs (VA) health care. Public Health Rep. 2007;122(1):93–100.
31. Bolouki A, Zal F. Impact of war on fertility and infertility. Arch Iran Med. 2020;23(4 Suppl 1):S16–22.
32. Katon JG, Zephyrin L, Meoli A, Hulugalle A, Bosch J, Callegari L, et al. Reproductive health of women veterans: a systematic review of the literature from 2008 to 2017. Semin Reprod Med. 2018;36(6):315–22.
33. Gerber MR. Trauma-informed care of veterans. In: Gerber MR, editor. Trauma-informed health care approaches: a guide for primary care. Cham: Springer Nature Switzerland AG; 2019. p. 107–22.
34. Martini AE, Doyle JO. Fertility preservation before deployment: oocyte and sperm freezing in members of the active duty military. Semin Reprod Med. 2019;37(5–06):232–8.
35. Lawson AK, Zweifel JE, Klock SC. Blurring the line between life and death: a review of the psychological and ethical concerns related to posthumous-assisted reproduction. Eur J Contracept Reprod Health Care. 2016;21(5):339–46.

Index

A
Acculturation process, 120
Active-duty military personnel, 130
Adopting practices, 86
Adverse childhood events (ACEs), 56, 69, 129
Adverse Childhood Experiences Questionnaire for Adults (ACEs), 88
Alleged medical fraud by fertility physicians, 44
Allies, 78
American College of Obstetricians and Gynecologists (ACOG), 31, 48, 62
American Journal of Obstetrics and Gynecology, 60
American Psychiatric Association, 55
American Society for Reproductive Medicine (ASRM), 2, 17–18, 59, 115, 123
Anatomical dissection, 72
Anesthesia ineffectiveness, 43
Aneuploid embryos, 86
Asherman's syndrome, 44
Assigned Female At Birth (AFAB), 54
Assigned Male At Birth (AMAB), 54
Assisted reproductive technologies, 58–59, 115, 133
Aversive conditioning, 55
Aversive reproductive experiences, 10
Avoidance-based reactions to trauma stimuli and distressing reactions, 31
Avoidance of gendered language, 61
Avoidance of healthcare, 57

B
Baby Boomer generation, 53
Biochemical pregnancy losses, 17, 86
Biological and genetic similarity, 68
Birth trauma, 44
Black and Brown bodies for medical experimentation, 71
Black, Indigenous, or People of Color (BIPOC), 70
Bladder washing with caustic solutions, 55
Burnout
  and compassion fatigue, 96, 97
  healthcare professionals and staff, 6
  primary causes, 2

C
Center for Health Care Strategies, 108
Center for Medicare and Medicaid Services, 56
Centers for Disease Control and Prevention, 53
Cervical cancer screening, 61
Chronic illnesses, 44
Chronic pain, medical issue, 44
Civilian medical care, 132
Clinic administrators and staff, strategies, 102–108, 110, 111
Clinic transparency and accountability, 47
Clinical pregnancies, 18
Clinic-approved egg and sperm banks, 79

A. Lawson, A. Swanson (eds.), *Trauma-Informed Reproductive Healthcare*, https://doi.org/10.1007/978-3-031-67474-7

Collaboration and mutuality, 49, 89, 90
Collaborative care, 76
Combat, 132
Combat fatigue, 3
Combat medicine and protective gear, 133
Compassion fatigue, 6, 9
Complex Racial Trauma (CoRT), 70
Complex trauma, 69
  exposure in childhood, 69
Contradictory research, 46
Conversion therapy, 55, 56
Coping mechanisms of reproductive medicine, 119
Cultural and religious beliefs, 76
Cultural competence, 75
Cultural humility, 75
Culturally-informed providers, 76

D
Deemed fertility fraud, 44
Diagnostic and Statistical Manual of Mental Disorders-5th edition (DSM-5), 3, 4, 31
Diagnostic and Statistical Manual-II (DSM-II), 55
Disclosure of traumatic experiences, 32
Discrimination, 10
  based on overweight/obesity, 43
Disenfranchised trauma, 41
Disparate access to care, 10
Distraction techniques, 21
DNA testing, 45
Doctor-patient conversation, 105

E
Early miscarriage, 92
Early pregnancy loss (EPL), 19, 20, 26
Ectopic pregnancies, 17, 42
Educating reproductive medicine teams, 119
Education and training on trauma and trauma-informed care, 106
Educational workshops on trauma-informed care to reproductive medicine clinics, 119
Egg retrieval, 44
Ego-dystonic homosexuality, 55
Electroconvulsive therapy, 55
Embedded and consultative MHPs, 124
Embedded support groups, 49
Embryo transfer procedures, 42
Emotional and physical trauma, 56, 58
Emotional distress, 119
Emotional dysregulation, 117
Emotional reactions, 85
Empathic social support, 10
Empirically supported implementation of trauma-informed care, 85
Empirically validated questionnaires, 87
Employee assistance program, 121
Employee recruitment and hiring process, 103, 104
Empowerment, 7, 90
  focused delivery of medical care, 131
  voice, and choice, 49
Ethnicity, 68

F
Failed embryo transfers, 17, 86
Failed fertilization/embryos, 86
Fears of discrimination, 57
Fears of stigma, 57
Fertility
  chronic illnesses, 44
  care, 43, 88, 92
  clinics, 48, 58, 116, 118
  clinics with medical trauma, 45
  counseling, 116, 125
  fraud, 10, 44
  and REI teams, trauma, 9
  treatment, 86
Fertility-related support groups, 123
Fetishism, 55
First Responders, 131
First Responders and military personnel, 130
Freud, Sigmund, 55

G
Gamete cryopreservation, 133
Gamete disposition, 133
Gamete donors, 133
  and gestational carriers, 123, 124, 133
  and surrogacy candidates, 123
Gate-keeper, 123
Gender, 53, 54
  expression, 53, 54
  identity, 53, 54
Gender-inclusive language, 60
Gender/sex binary, 60
Generation Z, 53
Genital dysphoria, 59
Genuine empathy, 123
Gestational carrier, 44
Government-sponsored sterilization of Black women in the South, 72
Grave robbers, 72
Gynecological and fertility procedures, 42

H
Health and psychosocial problems, 130
Health and wellness, 110, 111
Healthcare professionals, 87
  lived experiences, 87, 88
  and staff schedules, 104
Healthcare systems, 119–121
Homosexuality, 55
Hormonal transitions, psychotropic medications, 122
Hypervigilance, 43
Hypnosis, 55

I
Implementation coaching, 107
Implicit biases, 77
  in fertility care, 77, 78
Infertility, 10, 86
  and assisted reproductive technologies, 122
  and fertility preservation, 1
  participation in assisted reproduction, 118
  and pregnancy loss, 10
  psychological comorbidities, 115
Institutional accountability, 76
Institutional betrayal, 40, 43
Integrated mental health professionals, 11
Intensive Care Unit (ICU) stay, 41
Interpersonal violence (IPV), 61
  prevalence, 61
Intersectionality in health disparities research, 54
Intimate partner violence (IPV), 61
Intraoperative awareness, 41, 43
Intrauterine insemination, 42

L
Late-term pregnancy losses, 23, 24, 26
Legal protections, 59
LGBTQ+ (lesbian, gay, bisexual, transgender, queer) community
  2022 national survey, 53
  augmenting medical care, 57
  clinical practice, 58
  experienced/feared discrimination, 57
  health care, 57
  heterosexuality and gender binary, 53
  intake forms, 60
  interpersonal violence (IPV) survivors, 58
  knowledge and inclusivity, 60
  language, 60
  medical environment, 57
  medical marginalization, 59
  reproductive setting, 62
  visibility and acceptability, 53
LGBTQ-specific patient education, 60
Lifelong learning, 97
Lobotomies, 55

M
Medicaid, 108
Medical abuse, 40, 43
Medical and social discrimination/harassment, 42
Medical care, 39
  REI clinics, 8
  team, 87
Medical complications, 46
Medical cynicism, 43
Medical diagnoses, procedures and treatment, 39
Medical discrimination and microaggressions, 42
Medical errors in lab, 46, 47
Medical events, 45
Medical experimentation, 72
Medical forms, 60
Medical histories and consent forms, 88
Medical insurance benefits, 132
Medical marginalization, 62
Medical mistrust, 39
Medical perspective, 44
Medical prejudice and discriminatory practices, 59
Medical professionals, 87
Medical records, 132
Medical staff and healthcare professionals, 6
Medical team's competency, 43
Medical trauma
  assault/discrimination, 40
  direct contact with medical setting, 40
  discrimination and/or institutional betrayal, 40
  during fertility treatment, 44
  ethical and practice standards, 40
  fertility patients, 41
  fertility treatment, 41, 47
  history, 39
  medical errors, 40
  medical experiences, 40
  medical procedures/events, 41
  medical/surgical complications, 45
  painful transvaginal exams/ultrasounds, 45
  patient-provider relationship, 40
  personal experience, 45
  rates and prevalence, 41
  risk of, 9
  sense of trust and safety, 40
  sexual behaviors, 41
  types, 42

Medical trust, 131
Mental and physical health benefits for patients, 33, 34
Mental health professionals (MHPs), 11, 95
  mental health support, 122
  patient autonomy, 122
  psychosocial and neurobiological consequences of trauma, 117
Mental health resources, 122
Mental health services, 58
Mental health treatment, referrals to, 122
Military and first responder, 129, 132–135
Military service history, 131
Military sexual trauma (MST), 130
Minimal trauma, 86
Minor procedure and donor sperm, 45
Minoritized children, 69
Minoritized people in reproductive healthcare, 73–75
Minority stress theory, 54
Miscarriage, 17, 19, 21, 22
Mississippi appendectomy, 72
Mistaken belief, 73
Multiple pregnancy losses in woman, 18
Mutual learning and critical self-reflection, 75
Mutuality, 89

N
National Center for Trauma Informed Care's (NCTIC), 58
National Intimate Partner and Sexual Violence Survey (NISVS), 30, 56
National Study of Child Health, 69
2022 National Survey on LGBTQ Young Mental Health Survey, 56
National Violence Against Women Survey (NVAWS), 30
Needle and sedation exposure, 9
Non-clinically recognized reproductive losses, 26
Non-empathetic support from social networks and healthcare teams, 10
Nonjudgmental emotional support, 87
NSAID, 44

O
Obesity
  fertility clinics, 43
  infertility, 43
  intensive behavioral lifestyle changes, 43
  pregnancy loss, 43
ObGyns, 11, 34
Occupational aversive exposure, 3
Office of the National Coordinator of Health Information Technology, 56
Oocyte stimulation, 42
Organization/clinic-level policies and procedures, 102, 103
Organization's practice and procedural guidelines, 102
Ovarian torsion, 42

P
Pain tolerance of racialized people, 73
Pap tests, 59
Patient advocacy, 8
Patient advocacy staff members, 107
Patient appointment, 88
Patient care, 78–80
Patient empowerment, 122
Patient-provider relationship, 40
Pedophilia, 55
Peer support, 7, 12, 47, 49, 89
Penetrative intercourse, 59
Perinatal loss, 26
Personal reflection, 97
Physical and chemical castration, 55
Physical assault, 131
Physical conversion therapy methods, 55
Physical environment, 105, 106
Physiological arousal, 131
PLACE strategy, 78, 79
Planned and medical gamete cryopreservation, 86
Polyvictimization, 69
Posthumous reproduction, 133, 136
Postpartum psychosis, 122
Posttraumatic growth, 119
Posttraumatic stress disorder, 118
Pregnancy loss, 45, 46, 86
  early, 19, 20
Pregnancy loss, TIC
  emotional support from healthcare professionals, 24
  emotionally validating communication, 26
  fetal diagnosis, 25
  follow-up care after loss, 26
  harm and promote healing, 25
  incidence, 17
  perinatal loss, 24
  presumptive diagnosis, 18
  principles, 25
  psychological/lifestyle stress, 18
  psychological support services, 24
  strategies, 25

trauma-informed healthcare professionals, 25
treatment environment for patients, 24
types, 17
Pregnancy tests, negative, 86
Premenstrual dysphoric disorder, 123
Primary recurrent pregnancy loss, 18
Professional, empathic, evidence-based care, 24
Professional Quality of Life Scale (ProQOL), 110
Provider and staff schedules, 104
Provision of trauma-informed healthcare, 131
Psychiatric distress, 3
Psychoanalysis, 55
Psychological arousal, 131
Psychological assessment instruments, 124
Psychological distress, 3, 122
medication management, 122
screening, 11
Psychological reverberations, 18
Psychometric soundness, 117

Q

Qualified mental health professionals, 115, 116

R

Race and ethnicity, 68
chronic risk of exposure, 70
existence, 68
medical and health research, 68
migration experience, 69
minoritized identities, 69
minoritized populations, 69
physiological and psychological sequelae, 69
racialization of groups, 68
reporting, 68
social constructs, 68
sociodemographic factors and social determinants, 68
Race-based traumatic events, 70
Race-based traumatic stress, 69
Racial/ethnic category, 68
Racial trauma and medical system, 70–72
Rape, 30
Reciprocal/co-IVF for same-sex female patients, 59
Rectal massage, 55
Recurrent miscarriage, 18
Recurrent pregnancy loss (RPL), 20–22, 26
causes, 18
Red Scare anti-communist campaigns, 55
Re-labeling women's health clinics, 60
Reproductive capacity of Indigenous populations, 72
Reproductive care, 79
Reproductive care with ART for gender diverse patients, 59
Reproductive Endocrinology and Infertility (REI)
consultation, 93
setting, 129
teams, 7, 11
goals and resilience, 12
Reproductive Endocrinology and Infertility (REI) clinic, 1, 6, 7, 10, 86, 92
access to care and treatment outcomes, 8
cultural, historical and gender issues, 8
education, 12
errors, 10
highly distressed patient population, 8, 9
Reproductive endocrinology team, 86
Reproductive errors, 10
Reproductive futures, 34
Reproductive health outcomes, 58
Reproductive healthcare, 73
professionals, 131
providers, 58
Reproductive loss, 17, 24, 25
Reproductive medical care, 121
Reproductive medicine, 2, 85, 115, 116
Reproductive medicine clinics, 117
awareness of mental health referral options, 122
vaginal/internal exams and procedures, 34
Reproductive medicine patients with psychological distress, 118
Reproductive mental health professionals, contributions, 115
Reproductive psychiatry, 122
and psychotherapy, 123
Research on trauma-informed workplaces, 122
Resisting re-traumatization, 48
Respect and acknowledgement in cultural, historical, and gender issues, 49
Retrievals, 44

S

Sadism, 55
SAMHSA, *see* Substance Abuse and Mental Health Administration (SAMHSA)
Satisfaction absenteeism and intention, 31
Scheduling team, 94

Secondary recurrent pregnancy loss, 18
Secondary trauma
 burnout and compassion fatigue, 121
 clinic-wide trainings, 121
 physical, emotional, cognitive and behavioral symptoms, 121
 professional health, 121
 provider efficacy, 121
 on providers' professional and personal lives, 121
Self-care, 97
Self-discontinuation of psychotropic medications during fertility treatment, 122
Self-reflection, 12, 79
Servicemen's Readjustment Act of 1944, 55
Sex, 53
 assigned at birth, 54
 behavior, 9
Sexual and gender minority populations, 53
Sexual and reproductive health services, 60
Sexual assault, 30, 44
 and harassment, 30
Sexual orientation, 53, 54, 60
Sexual orientation disturbance, 55
Sexual victimization, 29, 31
 history, 32
 serious physical and psychological consequences, 31
 types, 30
Shared decision making, 12
Shell shock, 3
Social and health-related outcomes, 117
Social network, 25, 79
Social support, 10
Specialized trauma-informed medical and psychological care, 26
Spirituality, 120
Stigma, 10
Stigmatization/blame for traumatic event, 86
Stress, 35
Substance Abuse and Mental Health Administration (SAMHSA), 2, 4, 39, 58
 definition of trauma, 4
 model of trauma-informed care, 24
 National Center for Trauma-Informed Care, 108
 principal of Collaboration and mutuality, 7
Substance Abuse and Mental Health Administration's (SAMHSA) six key principles of TIC, 6, 86, 89
 examination/procedure, 48
 procedures/treatments, 48
 safety, 48
Supernumerary embryo disposition, 86
Supernumerary embryos, 17
Supportive conversation, 93
Supportive team environment, 110
Survival techniques, 118

T

Team support, 110
Telemedicine procedures, 106
Terminating a pregnancy due to fetal anomaly (TOPFA), 23, 24
Testicular implants, 55
Third-party reproduction, 76, 85, 123
 collaborator, 44
 psychological evaluations, 124
Title VI of the Civil Rights Act, 76
Trainings and certification on culturally modified psychotherapies, 121
Transparency, 7, 10, 48, 89, 92
Transparent and collaborative communication, 92
Transvaginal exams and ultrasounds, 45
Trauma
 concept of, 2
 exposure, 5
 screening, 11
 in written documentation, 11
Trauma exposure and psychological distress, 118
 interpersonal consequences, 118
 prevalence rates, 117
Trauma-informed care (TIC)
 application, 6
 cultural, historical, and gender issues, 90, 91
 healthcare team, 5
 medical and emotional risks, 5
 national importance and recognition, 2
 patient care, 5
 psychological distress, 35
 in reproductive medicine, 2
Trauma-informed delivery of bad news, 95, 96
Trauma-informed design, 105
Trauma-informed training to healthcare professionals, 117
Traumatic automobile accident, 131
Traumatic birth, 44
Traumatic events, prevalence, 4, 5

Traumatic pregnancy, 44
Trustworthiness, 7, 10, 48, 89
Tuskegee Study, 72

U
Underreporting of trauma, 130
Unexpected medical issues/diagnoses, 42
Unexpected surgical outcomes, 42
United States Centers for Disease Control and Prevention (CDC), 61
United States Supreme Court, 56
Universal screening of trauma in adult healthcare settings, 116, 117
Unwanted sexual contact violence, 30
US Department of Veterans Affairs, 134
U.S. National Intimate Partner and Sexual Violence Survey, 5

V
Value conflicts, 120
Verbal abuse, 43
Veteran Affairs (VA)
  health care settings, 132
  health care system, 55, 132
Veteran status, 131
Veteran's health, 133
Vicarious trauma, 6, 96, 108
  and compassion fatigue, 109
  education and assessment, 109, 110
  and increased stress levels, 109
  and stress, 109
Vicarious traumatization, 9, 107, 108
Victim-blaming, 10
  avoidance, 34
Victimization, allegations, 130
Voice and choice, 7

W
Wave 3 National Epidemiologic Survey on Alcohol and Related Conditions (NESARC-III), 130
Weight bias, 43
Women's Experience of Pain, 10
Workplace sexual harassment, 30
World Health Organization (WHO), 30